MICROBIOLOGY RESEARCH ADVANCES

ANIMAL MODELS IN CANCER RESEARCH AND HUMAN DISEASE

APPLICATIONS, OUTCOMES AND CONTROVERSIES

Microbiology Research Advances

Additional books in this series can be found on Nova's website
under the Series tab.

Additional e-books in this series can be found on Nova's website
under the e-book tab.

Animal Science, Issues and Professions

Additional books in this series can be found on Nova's website
under the Series tab.

Additional e-books in this series can be found on Nova's website
under the e-book tab.

MICROBIOLOGY RESEARCH ADVANCES

ANIMAL MODELS IN CANCER RESEARCH AND HUMAN DISEASE

APPLICATIONS, OUTCOMES AND CONTROVERSIES

SEAN A. MURRAY
EDITOR

New York

For permission to use material from this book please contact us:
Telephone 631-231-7269; Fax 631-231-8175
Web Site: http://www.novapublishers.com

Additional color graphics may be available in the e-book version of this book.

Library of Congress Cataloging-in-Publication Data

ISBN: 978-1-62417-587-9

Library of Congress Control Number: 2012954583

Published by Nova Science Publishers, Inc. † New York

Contents

Preface

This book discusses the applications, outcomes and controversies of using animal models in cancer research and human disease. Topics include murine models of sporadic and inflammation-related colon carcinogenesis with particular focus on the AOM/DSS chemically induced colorectal cancer model; large animal models of human cardiovascular disease; developments of cell therapeutic strategies for Alzheimer's disease using animal models; the techniques and limitations of murine models of human colorectal cancer; animal models for antineoplastic chemotherapy-induced alopecia; and development of columnar-lined esophagus with or without goblet cells in rate duodengastroesophageal reflux models through gut regenerative cell lineage (GRCL).

Chapter I – Colorectal cancer (CRC) is the third most common malignancy in the world. It is a life-threatening disease that can develop spontaneously or as a long-term complication of an inflammatory status. Inflammation can indeed provide initiating and promoting stimuli and mediators, generating a tumour-prone microenvironment. Although inflammation-linked carcinogenesis is a well accepted concept and is often observed within the gastrointestinal tract, the underlying mechanisms remain to be elucidated. Furthermore, the risk for CRC is also influenced by a genetic predisposition, which is especially high for somatic mutations of the tumor suppressor gene adenomatosis polyposis coli (APC), causing familial adenomatosis coli. Animal models are essential tools for the understanding of human CRC and for the preclinical testing of novel therapeutic options *in vivo*. Many murine models of sporadic and inflammation-related colon carcinogenesis have been developed in the last decade, including chemically induced CRC models, genetically engineered mouse models, and xenoplants. Although none of these models reflects all aspects of CRC, they complement each other to provide suitable tools for specific tasks. In this chapter, the authors discuss the principal features of different CRC models, considering they own benefits and limits. Then they will focus their attention on the chemically-induced CRC murine models reported in the literature as highly valuable and powerful model systems. Among them, the azoxymethane/dextran sodium sulphate (AOM/DSS) murine model is considered as a reliable practical tool, since the tumor development is predictable and consistent, with a high incidence of affected animals in a narrow time frame. More importantly, this model reproduces many aspects of human CRC development and it offers the possibility to study the earliest succession of events underlying tumor initiation, when single aberrant crypts appear in colonic mucosa. For this reason, the AOM/DSS model has become an outstanding model for studying the early molecular events, still partially unknown in humans, that act in the preneoplastic phase of colon carcinogenesis and which are fundamental in CRC development, representing a powerful platform also useful in

intervention studies.

Chapter II – In most countries, cardiovascular disease is one of the leading causes of death. The treatment and management of cardiovascular disease has advanced over the past 2 decades, largely due to the use of experimental animal models. Although a large amount of information can be generated with the use of experimental animal models, non-human animal models cannot fully replicate the complexity of human pathological conditions. Thus, a deeper understanding of the differences and similarities between humans and each animal model is important in preclinical research. Small animal models provide insight into the molecular and cellular basis of cardiovascular biology, but significant differences exist with regard to cardiovascular characteristics between small animal models and humans. Large animal models which simulate human cardiovascular physiology, anatomy and function are also crucial to develop clinical therapies and interventions. Here, the authors will mainly focus on the large animal models of cardiovascular disease, including coronary artery disease, heart failure, peripheral artery disease and structural heart disease.

Chapter III – While tumors in companion animals (dogs and cats) draw attention in the realm of pet care, they also offer unique opportunities to develop valid models in which to study human cancers and translational cancer therapeutics. Spontaneous tumors in dogs are appropriate intermediate model systems for a number of reasons. Dogs represent an out-bred population that has a shared environment with humans. Canine cancers often demonstrate similar histopathologic and biologic behavior to tumors occurring in humans, and the size of the model allows for extrapolation to humans. Canine mammary carcinoma and lymphoma are two excellent examples of tumors that have potential relevance to human cancer biology. Canine malignant mammary tumors are very common in middle aged, sexually intact female dogs and have a metastatic pattern similar to that in women. Moreover, mammary carcinomas in female dogs provide a high level of similarity in genetics, pathology and environmental exposure when compared to human breast cancer. Like humans, expression of canine cell proliferation and cell cycle regulatory genes are frequently altered in breast cancer. Lymphoma is a highly aggressive disease of dogs and is one of the most common tumors seen in the domestic dog. Middle-to-old age dogs are more often affected, with certain breeds showing increased incidence. The most common clinical presentation in dogs is similar to non-Hodgkin's lymphoma (NHL) in humans and as such has been proposed as a model for human disease. This canine model is further supported by the presence of evolutionarily conserved cytogenetic changes. Adding to the power of both canine breast cancer and lymphoma is the high similarity between dog and human genomes, allowing comparative genomics approaches to understanding these tumors and potential response to therapy.

Chapter IV – Alzheimer's disease (AD) is characterized by progressive cognitive impairment as a consequence of extensive neuronal loss. Pathological hallmarks of AD include the development of senile plaques formed by the accumulation of extracellular amyloid-β(Aβ) and neurofibrillary tangles (NFTs) consisting of intraneuronal accumulation of hyperphosphorylated tau. According to the amyloid cascade hypothesis, the accumulation of Aβin the brain parenchyma is the early event that influences other AD pathologies. Therefore, the reduction of brain Aβhas been considered a primary therapeutic target for AD. Since familial AD-linked genes have been found, many transgenic mouse models have been established and utilized in the experimental studies to examine the accuracy of amyloid cascade hypothesis and therapeutic strategies. In the studies, microglial phagocytosis has been noted as an Aβclearance system in the brain. Interestingly, microglia exogenously administered also affect the clearance of Aβ. In this context, cell therapeutic strategies aiming at replenishment of microglia-dependent functions in the brain have been proposed and the feasibility is about to be examined in the experimental study using transgenic mouse models of AD. In this chapter, the authors focused on cell therapeutic strategies, which have been constructed by the microglial beneficial functions, then summarized the current status of the studies. Experimental evidence hopefully suggest that the cell-based therapeutic approach could be a powerful strategy for AD treatment.

Chapter V – One of the most common and distressing side effects of cancer therapy is chemotherapy-induced alopecia (CIA). Approximately 65% of patients receiving anti-neoplastic therapies experience some degree of alopecia. The study of CIA had been hampered by the lack of suitable animal models; in this regard, the first animal models used to study CIA were impractical and difficult to extrapolate to the humans. In recent years, the development of the young rat models and the mouse model of CIA opened new avenues to the investigation and understanding of the mechanisms of CIA. However, there has been much controversy as to which model is more suitable to study the histopathology and molecular mechanisms of CIA. The young rat model has been employed due to the fact that 100% of the pelage hair follicles are in the growth phase during postnatal morphogenesis, therefore mimicking the human scalp where 90% of the hair follicles are undergoing anagen (active growth phase of the hair cycle) at any given time. In contrast, in the adult mouse and rat models, anagen synchronization needs to be induced by depilation or shaving to mimic the human scalp. These models have been extensively used in the search for protective agents against CIA. In this chapter, the authors will compare and contrast the different models and review the state-of-the-art findings in terms of animal models and protective agents.

Chapter VI – Murine models of colon carcinogenesis are an essential tool in understanding the mechanisms of pathogenesis and to evaluate therapeutic and preventive measures. Over the years considerable changes in the understanding of the murine models of human colon cancer has resulted in numerous models being reported in the literature. The reports of colon cancer transgenic mice were followed by human xenograft heterotopic murine models. With the orthotopic tumor models being found to be more relevant in portraying the human disease process as opposed to heterotopic models, many techniques for making orthotopic colorectal murine models were reported. Although all of these models have their advantages and limitations, the latest orthotopic murine models seem to accurately represent and replicate the human disease process. The authors discuss the different human colon cancer murine models, their background, the technique of creating them along with their advantages and limitations. This extensive overview and details of an array of different resources in this field offers the researchers a wide choice to choose a model which is more applicable to the type of study being planned.

Commentary – Previous studies have focused on goblet cells as the primary marker for Barrett's esophagus (BE), however, recently non-goblet cells, which are columnar-lined esophageal cells resembling gastric cardia-type mucosa, have also been used to define this disease. On the basis of results using rat gastroduodenal contents reflux models, many groups have demonstrated that BE-originating cells are derived from the transcommitment of the esophageal squamous progenitor cells. However, two different lines of evidence have been reported that challenge the transcommitment hypothesis. One is that a discrete population of residual embryonic cells, existing at the gastroesophageal junction in normal individuals, expands and migrates into the esophageal epithelium. The other is that BE originates from gastric cardia progenitors. Recently, the authors were able to induce cardia-type mucosa without goblet cells in a novel rat reflux model that mimics the human gastroduodenal reflux mechanism. In this the cardia-type mucosa originated not from cells located in the basal layer of the squamous epithelium but from the glandular stomach site. The cardia-type mucosa may progress to specialized intestinal metaplasia (SIM) following continuous bile acids exposure. The concentration and composition of bile acids in the reflux contents may be important factors to decide the pathway and phenotypic switch from gastric to intestinal. The authors found a peculiar metaplastic change and propose the concept GRCL:Gut regenerative cell lineage (GRCL) develops in response to chronic inflammation. This change is characterized by pyloric–foveolar metaplasia followed by the appearance of goblet cells. SIM also develops through GRCL.

In: Animal Models in Cancer Research ... ISBN: 978-1-62417-587-9
Editor: Sean A. Murray

Chapter I

Murine Models of Sporadic and Inflammation-Related Colon Carcinogenesis with Particular Focus on the AOM/DSS Chemically Induced Colorectal Cancer Model

***M. De Robertis*[1,2], *V. M. Fazio*[1,3] *and E. Signori*[1,2*]**

[1]Laboratory of Molecular Medicine and Biotechnology, CIR, University Campus Bio-Medico of Rome, Rome, Italy
[2]Laboratory of Molecular Pathology and Experimental Oncology, CNR-IFT, Rome, Italy
[3]Laboratory of Oncology, IRCCS 'Casa Sollievo della Sofferenza, 'San Giovanni Rotondo (FG), Italy

Abstract

Colorectal cancer (CRC) is the third most common malignancy in the world. It is a life-threatening disease that can develop spontaneously or as a long-term complication of an inflammatory status. Inflammation can indeed provide initiating and promoting stimuli and mediators, generating a tumour-prone microenvironment. Although inflammation-linked carcinogenesis is a well accepted concept and is often observed within the gastrointestinal tract, the underlying mechanisms remain to be elucidated. Furthermore, the risk for CRC is also influenced by a genetic predisposition, which is especially high

* Corresponding author: Dr Emanuela Signori, CNR-IFT, Laboratory of Molecular Pathology and Experimental Oncology, Area Ricerca Tor Vergata, Via Fosso del Cavaliere 100, 00133 Rome, Italy. E-mail: emanuela. Signori@ift.cnr.it.

for somatic mutations of the tumor suppressor gene adenomatosis polyposis coli (APC), causing familial adenomatosis coli.

Animal models are essential tools for the understanding of human CRC and for the preclinical testing of novel therapeutic options *in vivo*. Many murine models of sporadic and inflammation-related colon carcinogenesis have been developed in the last decade, including chemically induced CRC models, genetically engineered mouse models, and xenoplants. Although none of these models reflects all aspects of CRC, they complement each other to provide suitable tools for specific tasks.

In this chapter, we discuss the principal features of different CRC models, considering they own benefits and limits. Then we will focus our attention on the chemically-induced CRC murine models reported in the literature as highly valuable and powerful model systems. Among them, the azoxymethane/dextran sodium sulphate (AOM/DSS) murine model is considered as a reliable practical tool, since the tumor development is predictable and consistent, with a high incidence of affected animals in a narrow time frame. More importantly, this model reproduces many aspects of human CRC development and it offers the possibility to study the earliest succession of events underlying tumor initiation, when single aberrant crypts appear in colonic mucosa. For this reason, the AOM/DSS model has become an outstanding model for studying the early molecular events, still partially unknown in humans, that act in the preneoplastic phase of colon carcinogenesis and which are fundamental in CRC development, representing a powerful platform also useful in chemo preventive intervention studies.

Keywords: Colorectal Carcinogenesis; AOM/DSS Murine Model; Chemical Carcinogenesis; Colorectal Cancer Animal Models

Introduction

Colorectal cancer (CRC) is the third most common malignant neoplasm according to prevalence and mortality in the Western world. Worldwide, colorectal cancer represents 9.4% of all incident cancer in men and 10.1% in women, with just over 1 million new cases recorded in 2002, the most recent year for which international estimates are available [1]. It can develop spontaneously or as a late complication of chronic environmental stimuli. Predisposition to CRC is influenced by both environmental and genetic factors. For example, many environmental causes of cancer and other risk factors are associated with some form of chronic inflammation. Up to 20% of cancers are linked to chronic infections, 30% can be attributed to tobacco smoking and inhaled pollutants (such as silica and asbestos), and 35% can be attributed to dietary factors (for example, 20% of the cancer burden is linked to obesity). Importantly, CRC may arise as a long-term complication of inflammatory bowel disease (IBD), including ulcerative colitis (UC) and Crohn's disease (CD) [2].

Furthermore, the development of CRC can be influenced by genetic predisposition. Approximately 15-30% of all CRC cases show familial clustering of which only up to 5% can be explained by inherited mutations, mostly in the tumor suppressor gene adenomatosis polyposis (APC), that causes familial adenomatosis coli syndrome, or the mismatch repair genes (MMR-genes), the hallmark of Hereditary Nonpolyposis Colorectal Cancer (HNPCC) [3]. The 8-9% of CRC arises sporadically. Sporadic CRC develops through aberrant crypt foci (ACF) and adenomatous polyps from normal colonic epithelial cells, caused by accumulation of mutations in the tumor suppressor genes APC, SMAD4, DCC and p53 and the oncogene K-Ras. For the remaining familial CRC cases the underlying genetics remains elusive [4].

A variety of available CRC animal models have provided important tools for investigating the complex development and pathogenesis of CRC. Although none of the available models of CRC reflects etiology and pathobiology of human tumors in its entirety, both *in vitro* and *in vivo* models are available to reflect every stage of CRC development. These models are not only precious instruments for uncovering new mechanisms of CRC pathophysiology but are also promising tools for advancing our understanding of the tumor response to novel chemopreventive and therapeutic strategies.

There are numerous CRC animal models that can be opportunely used in preclinical studies so that human diagnostic- and therapeutics-oriented trials can become more focused, with greater chances of success. Each model displays its own peculiar advantages and limitations, thus, any specific experimental issue should be studied by choosing the model best suited to resolve particular tasks.

In this chapter, we describe different rodent models developed in the last few years for the study of CRC, with an extensive overview of the currently most commonly used model of chemically induced colon carcinogenesis, the AOM/DSS model, based on Azoxymethane/ Dextran Sodium Sulfate treatment. Here we compare the different protocols of tumor induction, present a comprehensive description of the histopathologic and molecular features of the AOM/DSS model and discuss its main advantages and limitations, as well as its recent experimental applications.

A Variety of CRC Models: Benefits and Limits

CRC development is a long-term process, from normal epithelial cells via aberrant crypts and progressive adenoma stages to carcinomas *in situ* and then metastases. A variety of models of CRC have been developed that mimic the etiology and pathobiology of human tumors; both *in vitro, in vivo* and *in silico* models can reflect every stage of CRC development. They are listed below highlighting peculiar benefits and limits.

In vitro models: a multitude of well-characterized CRC cell lines provide a wide spectrum of defined tumor cells displaying characteristic mutations, gene expression patterns and growth characteristics.

In vitro models permit isolation of specific aspects of tumor biology such that functional analysis of relevant genes and the assessment of effects of endogenous mediators and pharmacological compounds are faster and simpler than in the intact organism. Furthermore, most CRC cell lines grow rapidly in standard media and can easily be transfected to overexpress or knockdown key genes.

However, *in vitro* models can reflect only specific stages of tumor development, depending on the stage they have originated from. For cell lines this restricts the model to tumor stages with sufficient intrinsic growth potential, that is, carcinomas and with much more difficulty adenomas. Adenoma cells have less intrinsic growth potential so that their maintenance is more difficult than for carcinoma cell lines, requiring defined media and careful passaging [5].

In contrast, primary cultures can be produced from cells at all stages of tumor development in rodents and humans, and retain growth control and cellular interactions like *in vivo*. They reflect the same stage features of the tumor of origin, permitting direct comparisons and application of the results to the *in vivo* situation. However, they frequently provide only little material and are difficult to maintain especially where normal cells are concerned.

Finally, a major disadvantage of *in vitro* models, when investigating a complex disease like CRC, is the loss of tissue context that affects tumor growth and metastases *in vivo*.

In vivo models: many rodent models have been developed to evaluate various features of the carcinogenesis or metastatic process as seen in human CRC. Some of these models date back almost 80 years. Oncogenesis studies using these models have elucidated the role of genetic and environmental factors and of other influences on the various aspects of this complex disease, providing precious information on the initiation, promotion, and progression of tumors. The established models are currently used for chemoprevention studies as well as to evaluate immunological, chemical, and surgical therapy regimens.

Rodent models of CRC may be classified in three different groups a) genetically modified animals; b) xenoplant models; c) chemically-induced models.

a) Genetic models: the most common example of these models is represented by the Min/ΔAPC-mouse strains, which reproduce tumor development starting from initiated (mutated) epithelial cells to cover polyp growth through tumor progression and, rarely, metastases. Mutant mice carry a heterozygous germ line mutation in the APC gene (Min/ΔAPC-mouse), similar to that found in familial adenomatous polyposis (FAP) patients [6]. These animals develop multiple intestinal neoplasia (Min-mouse); they mimic the rapid tumor development seen in FAP patients and model the process of polyp growth and progression.

The one striking difference between Min/ΔAPC-mice and human FAP patients is tumor location, which is predominately in the small intestine and extremely rare in the colon of Min-mice, whereas, by contrast, FAP patients while also developing small intestinal tumors, carry large numbers of adenomatous polyps in their colon and rectum.

In the tumors, the loss of the APC allele, which normally prevents binding and degradation of β-catenin, constitutively activates the Wnt-pathway and deregulates growth in tumor cells. K-Ras mutations and inactivation of p53 have not been observed in Min-mouse tumors.

Different ΔAPC-mouse strains have been used for functional analysis of the APC gene product and mapping of essential domains. In addition, double mutant mouse strains have been constructed that carry both a mutated APC gene and alterations in modifier genes. For example, mice with homozygous deletions of phospholipase A2, [7] cyclooxygenase-2 (COX-2), [8] and prostaglandin-receptors EP2 and EP4 [9] present impaired neovascularisation of polyps and attenuated tumor development, which has also been observed in human colorectal polyps. Inactivation of Smad3, a frequent defect in human CRC, causes accelerated tumorigenesis and metastases to the lymph nodes [10].

Min-mouse models are widely used in the search for nutritional risk factors and chemopreventive compounds, usually by adding the test compound to the animal's diet.

Construction of mouse models for hereditary nonpolyposis colorectal cancer (HNPCC) has been less successful as the heterozygous deletion of the mismatch repair genes involved (Msh2, Mlh1, Msh6, Msh3, Pms2, and Pms1) did not prove to be sufficient to predispose to cancer. Consequently, mice carrying homozygous deletions have been used as disease models for HNPCC-like cancers [10]. Although such mice are more susceptible to tumor formation, the tumor spectrum observed consists of various lymphomas that are almost never encountered in HNPCC affected patients. Gastrointestinal tumors are only observed in animals that do not succumb to lymphomas in early life. Deletions in Msh2 and Pms2 potentiate APC-mediated intestinal tumorigenesis [10].

b) Xenoplant models: the ability of tumor cells to develop tumors after subcutaneous or intravenous injection in immunodeficient mouse strains (nude, bg/nu/xid, or SCID mice), allows the analysis of human tumors *in vivo* [11]. The xenoplant model reflects tumor growth and metastasis. As it is straightforward and easily achievable, it has been used to supply human tumors in an experimental *in vivo* environment for the assessment of cytostatic therapeutic compounds. Although the introduction of xenoplant models represents an important step towards a pathobiologically relevant model of tumor metastasis, xenoplants are only feasible using malignant cells that have sufficient intrinsic growth potential to form tumors in animal hosts, moreover subcutaneous or intravenous injections of tumor cells establish a model that neglects the complexity of tumor growth and metastasis and the interactions between tumor and microenvironment, which largely controls the biological characteristics of tumors. Orthotopic transplantation into the cecum and rectum has been developed to overcome this problem and creates a clinically accurate model for human CRC. From orthotopically-transplanted tumors, metastases spread to local lymph nodes and liver as expected [12]. However, an important practical limit of orthotopical transplant is the complexity of the surgical procedure involved, along with the lack of immune function that is a necessary element of all xenoplant models. These limitations eliminate the principal mechanisms that govern the effects of inflammation and immunity on tumor development.
c) Chemically-induced models: carcinogen-induced colon cancer in rodents can recapitulate in a highly reliable way the phases of initiation and progression of tumors that occur in humans. Chemical induction of tumors acts on the normal epithelium to form carcinomas via the classical multistage process of colon carcinogenesis but only rarely yields metastases. Such models are frequently used to assess the activity of chemopreventive compounds and to identify risk factors. Even if the high carcinogen dose given in experimental settings differs from the common situation in humans, where tumors arise from exposure to small doses of carcinogen present in the typical Western-style diet plus additional environmental factors, there are a number of advantages in studying the pathogenesis of carcinogen-induced colon cancer in rodents. These models are highly reproducible, they can be readily tested on animals with different genetic backgrounds, and the pathogenesis can recapitulate human CRC.

Of note is also the availability of *in silico* models, based on comparative analysis of gene expression, cancer chromosomes and mutations that have been performed by several groups in the last years. Individual studies searched for genes correlating with prognosis or therapy response as well as genes already expressed in adenomas. Data sets are available on-line, most prominently from the NCBI home page (http://www.ncbi.nlm.nih.gov/) and from the Johns Hopkins Oncology Center (http://www.sagenet.org) and can be used to identify tumor-specific alterations. However, *in silico* analysis of gene expression has so far remained isolated, and focused on specific single genes. A general meta-analysis of the available data that could provide an *in silico* model of colon cancer has not yet been performed.

Chemically Induced Colon Carcinogenesis in Rodents

A variety of chemical agents have been used to induce colon tumors in animals. They include direct- and indirect-acting agents, according to the requirement of biological catalysis to form the ultimate reactive species.

Table 1. Different rodent models based on chemical tumor induction of colorectal cancer

Carcinogen-induced models of sporadic CRC			
Chemical agents	Rodent strains	Treatment	Selected references
HETEROCYCLIC AROMATIC AMINES			
IQ (2-Amino-3-methylimidazo [4,5-f] quinoline)	F344 rats	IQ (125 ppm) in the diet for 58 wks.	Reddy et al., 1993 [11]
	SCID mice	IQ (300 ppm) in the diet for 32 wks.	Salim et al., [35]
	F344 rats	IQ (0.03%) in the diet for 14 wks.	Mølck et al., 2001 [36]
PhIP (2-Amino-1-methyl-6-phenylimidazol [4,5-b] pyridine)	F344 rats	PhIP (25 or 100 ppm) in the diet for up to 104 weeks.	Hasegawa et al., 1993 [10]
	F344 rats	PhIP (25, 100 or 400 ppm) in the diet for 48 wks.	Ito et al., 1997 [37]
	F344 rats	PhIP (50 mg/kg) oral gavage every day for 2 wks.	Wang et al., 2008 [38]
	F344 rats	3 cycles of 2-wk feeding PhIP (400 ppm) on basal diet with 4-wk intervals on high-fat diet without PhIP.	Nakagama et al., 2002 [39]
PhIP + AOM (Azoxymethane)	F344 rats	2 s.c. injections of AOM (15 mg/Kg bw) and	Doi et al., 2005 [12]

Carcinogen-induced models of sporadic CRC			
Chemical agents	Rodent strains	Treatment	Selected references
		various doses (0, 0.001, 0.01, 0.1, 1, 10, 50 and 200 ppm) of PhIP in the diet.	
DMABP (3,2'-Dimethyl-4-aminobiphenyl)	Albino rats	s.c. injections of DMABP (3.6-5.8 g/kg bw/day) for 131 or 376 days.	Walpole et al., 1952 [14]
	F344 rats	s.c. injections of DMABP (50 mg/kg bw/wk) for 20 wks.	Reddy et al., 1993 [15]
ALKYLNITROSAMIDE COMPOUNDS			
MNU (Methylnitrosourea)	Shrews	16 doses i.r. infusion of MNU (0.5-1.5 mg) administered biweekly.	Yang et al., 1996 [40]
MNNG (N-methyl-N'-nitro-N-nitrosoguanidine)	Sprague-Dawley rats	i.r. infusion of MNNG (2 mg/rat) twice a wk for 2 wks.	Zusman et al., 1991 [41]
	CD-Fischer rats	1 i.r. infusion of MNNG (4 mg/rat) + bile acids as tumor promoters.	Narisawa et al., 1974 [16]
DIMETHYLHYDRAZINE AND METABOLIC DERIVATIVES			
DMH (1,2-Dimethylhydrazine)	BD-IX rats	s.c. injections of DMH (15 mg/Kg bw) once a wk for 7 months.	Martin et al., 1973 [19]
	F344 rats	s.c. injections of DMH (26.6 mg/kg bw/wk) for 20 wks.	Ward et al., 1974 [20]
	Balb/c mice	s.c. injections of DMH (20 mg/kg bw/wk) for 10 wks.	Clapp et al., 1984 [27]
	SWR/J mice	i.p. injections of DMH (6.8 mg/kg bw/wk) for 1, 5, 10, or 20 wks.	Hata et al., 2004 [28]
AOM (Azoxymethane)	SWR/J, A/J mice	i.p. injections of AOM (10 mg/kg bw) for 6 or 8 wks.	Papanikolaou et al., 1998 [22] Papanikolaou et al., 2000 [23, 28]
	SWR/J, A/J mice	s.c. injections of AOM (15 mg/kg bw/wk) for 3 wks.	Hata et al., 2004 [28]
	AKR/J, C57BL/6J, DBA/2J, and SWR/J mice	i.p. or s.c. injections of AOM (5, 10, or 20 mg/kg bw) for 2, 4, or 8 wks.	Bissahoyo et al., 2005 [30]

Table 1. (Continued)

Carcinogen-induced models of sporadic CRC			
Chemical agents	Rodent strains	Treatment	Selected references
	FVB/N, 129/SvJ, C57Bl/6J mice A/J, AKR/J, Balb/CJ mice	i.p. injections of AOM (10 mg/kg bw) for 4 wks. i.p. injections of AOM (10 mg/kg bw) for 6 wks.	Nambiar et al., 2003 [42]
MODELS OF COLITIS-INDUCED CRC			
DSS (Dextran Sodium Sulfate)	C57Bl/6J mice	15 cycles of: 7 days 0.7% DSS followed by 10 days water.	Kim et al., 2010 [43]
Chemical agents	Rodent strains	Treatment	Selected references
	CBA/J mice	9 cycles of: 7 days 3% DSS followed by 14 days water.	Okayasu et al., 2002 [73]
	Swiss Webster mice	4 cycles of: 7 days 5% DSS followed by 14 days water.	Cooper et al., 2000 [53]
MODELS BASED ON COMBINATION OF CARCINOGEN AND PROINFLAMMATORY AGENT			
MeIQx, IQ, or PhIP + DSS	C57BL/6J mice	Diet containing MeIQx (300 ppm), IQ (300 ppm), or PhIP (300 ppm) for 12 wks followed by 2 cycles of 1-wk 1.5% DSS, 2 wks apart.	Nishikawa et al., 2005 [44]
DMH + DSS	Balb/c mice	1 i.p. injection of DMH (10-20 mg/kg bw) followed by 1-wk 2% DSS, after 1 wk from AOM.	Kohno et al., 2005 [54]
AOM + DSS	CBA/J mice FVB/N mice	1 i.p. injection of AOM (7.4 mg/kg bw) followed by 3 cycles of 1-wk 3% DSS (each cycle included of 3% DSS in drinking water for 7 days, followed by distilled water for 14 days).	Okayasu et al., 1996 [31] Becker et al., 2004 [32] Becker et al., 2005 [33]
	Balb/c, C3H/HeN, C57BL/6N and DBA/2N mice	1 i.p. injection of AOM (10 mg/kg bw), followed by 1% DSS for 4 days.	Suzuki et al., 2007 [46]
	Crj:CD-1 (ICR), Balb/c, C57Bl/6J mice	1 i.p. injection of AOM (10 mg/kg bw) followed by 1-wk 2% DSS, after 1 wk from AOM.	Tanaka et al., 2003 [24] Rosenberg et al., 2009 [34]

Abbreviations: s.c.: subcutaneous; i.p.: intraperitoneal; i.r.: intrarectal; bw: body weight; w/v: weight /volume; wk: week.

Unlike direct-acting agents, the indirect-acting carcinogens require enzymatic action to be converted into the active species which are able to alter cellular macromolecules such as nucleic acids or proteins.

Chemical carcinogens widely used to induce colon lesions similar to human malignancy, listed in Table 1, can be divided in the following categories: (a) heterocyclic aromatic amines, (b) alkylnitrosamide compounds, and (c) dimethylhydrazine and metabolic derivatives. The carcinogenic properties of these substances and their effects on histogenesis, cell proliferation kinetics, interaction between genetic susceptibility traits and environmental factors have been reported.

A. HETEROCYCLIC AROMATIC AMINES: heterocyclic amines (HCAs) and polycyclic aromatic hydrocarbons (PAHs) are chemicals formed during the cooking of meat and fish. In laboratory experiments, HCAs and PAHs have been found to be mutagenic and carcinogenic compounds, able to induce changes in DNA that may increase the risk of cancer.

   HCAs are formed when amino acids, sugars, and creatinereact at high temperatures. PAHs are formed when fat and juices from meat grilled directly over an open fire drip onto the fire, causing flames. These flames contain PAHs that then adhere to the surface of the meat. PAHs can also be formed during other food preparation processes, such as smoking of meats. PAHs can be found in other charred foods, as well as in cigarette smoke and car exhaust fumes.

   In many experiments, rodents fed a diet supplemented with HCAs developed tumors of the colon, but also to breast, liver, skin, lung, prostate, and other organs [13,14].

   Rodents fed PAHs also developed cancers of the gastrointestinal tract and lungs. However, the doses of HCAs and PAHs used in these studies were very high, equivalent to thousands of times the doses that a person would consume in a normal diet.

   The main representative carcinogens of the HCAs group, i.e., 2-amino-33-methylimidazo [4,5-f]quinoline (IQ) and 2-amino-1-methyl-6-phenylimidazol [4,5-b]pyridine (PhIP), have been introduced into experimental CRC. These compounds show a multi-target-organ specificity, with induction of lesions also in the mammary gland and prostate of rodents [15]. Liver metabolic activation of IQ to its ultimate carcinogen is required prior to IQ-DNA adduct formation which has been reported in different organs. Studies on PhIP activation and detoxification suggest that repeated exposures in colonic mucosa are required to activate PhIP *in vivo.* Dietary administration of IQ and PhIP in rodents for 52 weeks resulted in a low tumor incidence (5%–28%), [15] whereas with a PhIP-feeding regimen for 104 weeks [16] colon tumor incidence (43%–55%) was associated with severe toxicity. Moreover, combining PhIP with a high-fat diet or with AOM [17] causes enhancement of mutagenic and tumorigenic effects. PhIP induces a higher frequency of mutations in APC as well as microsatellite instability, but causes neither K-Ras nor p53 mutations [18].

   3,2'-dimethyl-4-aminobiphenyl (DMABP) is often used and similarly to other aromatic amine carcinogens, DMABP must be metabolically activated to exert its genotoxicity. This is accomplished via a multistep process leading to a final product that forms covalent adducts with DNA and this is thought to be a prerequisite for the initiation of the carcinogenic process. Chemical induction of both benign and malignant epithelial neoplasms in rat and in rodent models with (DMBA) has been described [19]. However, DMBA tumorigenic activity is less potent than that with the series of compounds derived from the other chemical carcinogens. For this reason, multiple injections of DMAB are required to induce colon tumors. There is also induction of neoplasms in other tissues [20].

B. ALKYLNITROSAMIDE COMPOUNDS: Methylnitrosourea (MNU) and N-methyl-N'-nitro-N-nitrosoguanidine (MNNG) are alkylating carcinogens that require an intrarectal injection to induce lesions in the distal colon and rectum in rodent models [21].

In rats and mice, most of the induced colonic tumors are sessile or polypoid lesions.

Because biochemical activation is not required, these compounds might be ideal topical carcinogens. On the other hand, the mode of administration represents their weakness.

It has been shown that intrarectal administration of MNNG at a dose rate of 1–3 mg/rat/week for 20 weeks induces colon tumors in 100% of male F344 rats, of which 43% tumors are adenocarcinomas and 57% are adenomas. The neoplasms are all located in the distal colon and rectum where MNNG and MNU are applied. The adenocarcinomas induced are mostly well-differentiated types with infiltration into the submucosa, whereas some are poorly differentiated showing mucinous cancer cells infiltrating into the submucosa. Metastases are not usually observed [22,18].

C. DIMETHYLHYDRAZINE AND METABOLIC DERIVATIVES: the most commonly used carcinogens for sporadic (non-familial) CRC models are 1,2-dimethylhydrazine (DMH) and its metabolite azoxymethane (AOM). Identification of these carcinogens arose initially from an early population study of Guamanians in which hydrazines were reported to be possible colon carcinogens. The hydrazine source was cycad flour eaten by this population. The carcinogen in cycad flour was found to be cycasin, a form of methylazoxymethanol (MAM), a downstream metabolite of DMH or AOM [23].

Repetitive treatment with this methylating agent was reported to produce colon tumors in rodents that exhibit many of the pathological features associated with the human disease [24,25]. Thus DMH has provided cancer researchers a reproducible experimental system for studying 'sporadic' forms of CRC.

Both DMH and AOM require several metabolic activation steps (including N-oxidation and hydroxylation) to induce DNA-reactive adducts. Hydroxylation of AOM results in the formation of the reactive metabolite MAM, which can alkylate macromolecules in the liver and colon, and operate the addition of methyl groups at the O6 or N7 position of guanine (O6-methyl-deoxyguanosine and N7-methyl-deoxyguanosine) in the DNA molecule. Methylation at the O6-position of guanine has been shown to be the primary promutagenic lesion produced by AOM. Other enzymes are involved in the metabolic activation of AOM. An *in vitro* study suggested that MAM activation in mouse is independent of colon alcohol dehyidrogenase [26]. On the other hand, the alcohol-inducible cytochrome P-450 isoform, CYP2E1, plays an important role in the conversion of AOM to MAM.

In the earliest published studies repetitive administration of DMH in rodents was demonstrated to induce colon tumors with pathological features similar to those observed in sporadic human disease [27,28]. Later studies switched to AOM [29,30], due to practical advantages such as reproducibility, enhanced potency, simple mode of application, great stability in dosing solution, and low price.

Numerous protocols with DMH or AOM, alone or in combination with DSS, have been used in different mice strains, based on repetitive administrations of only DMH or AOM, as well as colitis associated CRC models based on the AOM/DSS protocol.

- BALB/c mice treated with 10 subcutaneous (s.c.) injections of DMH (20 mg/kg body weight/week) and sacrificed 40 weeks after the first DMH injection have been shown to develop tumors with high incidence, almost exclusively in the distal colon [31].
- SWR/J mice treated with increasing intraperitoneal (i.p.) doses of DMH (6.8, 34, 68, and 136 mg/kg body weight) showed a dose-dependent decrease in survival time [32]. Four different protocols based on i.p. injections of DMH (6.8 mg/kg body weight/week) were tested, administering the carcinogen once a week for 1, 5, 10, or 20 weeks. At 20 weeks, colon tumors developed in 26%, 76%, and 87% of mice given a total dose of 34, 68, and 136 mg/kg DMH, respectively; no tumors were detected in animals treated with a total dose of 6.8 mg/kg. Most colon tumors (79%) were located in the distal colon, with the remainder being found in the mid-colon; no tumors were detected in either the proximal colon or the small intestine.
- SWR/J mice subjected to 3 s.c. injections of AOM (15 mg/kg body weight/week) and sacrificed at 35 weeks after the start of treatment have been reported to show a high incidence of colonic tumors [32]. Interestingly, although AKR/J mice had a lower incidence of colonic tumors at 35 weeks than SWR/J mice, the frequency of ACF was similar in AOM-treated AKR/J and AOM-treated SWR/J mice. In both strains, ACF were detected at high frequency in the proximal colon, whereas tumors arose mainly in the distal colon.
- A/J or SWR/J mice treated with 6 repeated i.p. injections of AOM (10 mg/kg body weight/week) and killed at 1, 2, 4, 6, 9, and 24 weeks after the last injection showed high incidence of colorectal tumors at week 24. Neoplasm formation could be revealed as early as 4 weeks after AOM exposure [33]. Bissahoyo *et al.* suggested that 4 injections might be sufficient for a high tumor induction rate (~90%) in the highly susceptible A/J strain but not in moderately susceptible ones such as the SWR/J strain [34].
- Female CBA/J subjected to 1 i.p. injection of AOM (7.4 mg/kg body weight) followed by three exposition cycles to DSS (each cycle included administration of 3% DSS in drinking water for 7 days, followed by distilled water for 14 days) showed a latency time of 12 weeks [35]. Multiple mucosal tumors (10.5/mouse) in combination with chronic colitis developed in the colorectum. More recently, similar results have been reported in FVB/N mice [36,37]. This model reproduces a state of

chronic inflammation, the driving force in tumor progression of colitis-associated CRC, as seen in UC or CD [30,35,36].

- Crj:CD-1 (ICR) mice (outbred strain) [29] receiving 1 i.p. injection of AOM (10 mg/kg body weight/week) followed by DSS (2%) in drinking water for 7 days (1 week after the AOM injection) showed 100% incidence of adenocarcinomas at 20 weeks after the first treatment, whereas another study revealed the presence of tumors already at week 6 [37]. Four other inbred murine strains (Balb/c, C57BL/6N, C3H/HeN, and DBA/2N) were used in the same experimental conditions. Among these, Balb/c mice displayed the same findings as was obtained with the ICR strain, whereas C57BL/6N, C3H/HeN, and DBA/2N were demonstrated to be more resistant to AOM. This last study demonstrated that when AOM is combined with the proinflammatory stimulus DSS, tumor growth is accelerated and there is a significantly shorter latency time (2–3 months).

The AOM/DSS Model in the Study of Colorectal Carcinogenesis

A number of experiments have demonstrated the relevance of the AOM/DSS mouse model in the study of the mechanisms of human colorectal carcinogenesis. Such model is particularly applicable when the focus of the study is on spontaneous tumor progression. Due to the synergic effects of AOM (tumor-inducing agent) and DSS (tumor-promoting agent), the AOM/DSS model reproduces colorectal carcinogenesis promoted by an initial acute inflammation phase, showing a shorter latency period than models based on only AOM or DSS administration. For instance, oral administration of a DSS solution to rodents, a widely used IBD mode, typically requires a long time exposure or many cycles of DSS administration and, moreover, the incidence of tumors is relatively low [30].

The AOM/DSS model offers relevant advantages in the study of CRC carcinogenesis when compared to the other chemical models previously described: tumor development is predictable and consistent, it requires a very simple mode of application, it displays a wide range of susceptibilities, and a high incidence of affected animals can be observed in a narrow time frame.

In the last year, two kinds of protocols based on AOM/DSS treatment have been developed.

The first is a two-stage AOM/DSS model (based on a single AOM injection followed by a cycle of DSS administration), which reproduces a tumor progression promoted by a short period of acute inflammation; the second is a four-stage protocol (based on three cycles of DSS administration, causing chronic colitis, in combination with the preceding single AOM injection) [31].

The two step model closely mirrors the pattern seen in human sporadic CRC. Tumors generated by AOM/DSS treatment accurately recapitulate the pathogenesis observed in humans. For example, tumors are very frequent in the distal part of the colon, which is also the predominant location of spontaneous CRC in man.

They often start with a polypoid growth and frequently exhibit histopathological features similar to human CRC. However, AOM-induced tumors often lack mucosal invasiveness.

Although AOM-induced colon tumors in mice and rats have a very low tendency to metastasize, the analysis of lymph nodes and other peripheral organs by macroscopic and microscopic techniques might be considered for studies examining factors potentially involved in metastasis.

The four step model represents a model of chronic inflammation which is believed to be the driving force in tumor progression of colitis-associated CRC, as seen in UC or CD [31].

As described by Tanaka *et al.* [29] the AOM/DSS model (two step model) is based on a single i.p. injection of AOM (10 mg/kg body weight) and a single cycle of the inflammatory agent DSS (2% weight/volume) in drinking water.

As shown in Figure 1, in this protocol there is a rapid development of multiple colon tumors in the outbred strain (crj:CD1) as well as in the inbred strain (Balb/c) within approximately 10 weeks [30].

DSS dissolved in drinking water is toxic to the epithelial lining of the colon and produces severe colitis, which is characterized by loss of body weight and bloody diarrhea in the first weeks following DSS consumption; however, these phenomena decrease significantly after 5 weeks from the start of AOM/DSS treatment.

AOM/DSS protocol is very reliable in inducing CRC with high penetrance and low mortality in highly susceptible mouse strains.

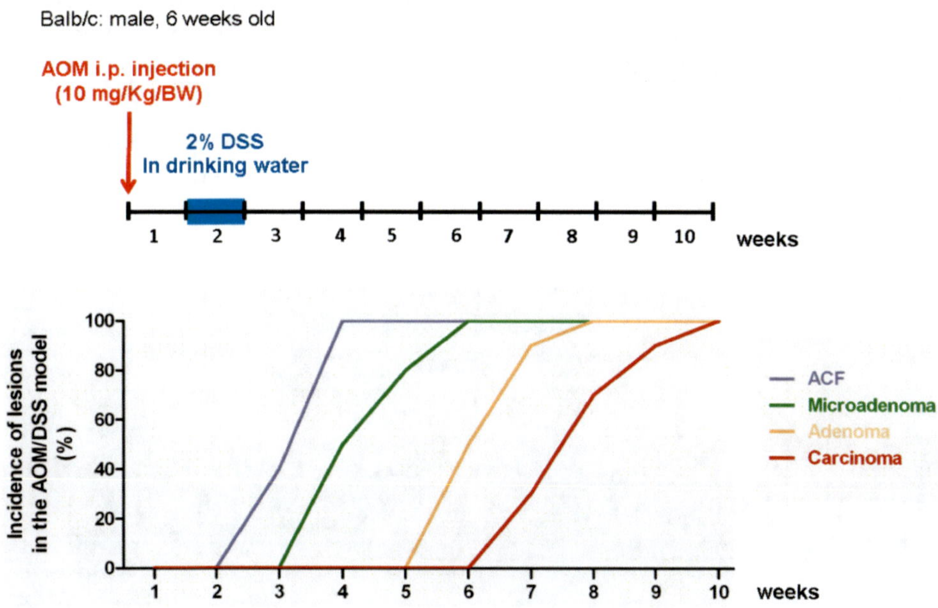

Figure 1. Experimental protocol of time-course observation of AOM/DSS-induced carcinogenesis in inbred Balb/c mice.

As in the human population, the genetic background of different rodent strains used to develop the AOM/DSS model, has been demonstrated to play an important role in the risk for colorectal tumorigenesis. After a first series of colon carcinogenesis studies in rats, in the last years the scientific community has largely switched to mouse models of CRC.

This is due to the advantages of murine models, such as the availability of extensive genetic information on individual mouse strains, the existence of recombinant inbred mouse panels, and the ever-increasing number of transgenic, knockout and knockin genetic models that are available for study.

Several studies to investigate the susceptibilities of different murine strains to AOM/DSS treatment have been conducted. Suzuki *et al.* [51] demonstrated differential sensitivities to the AOM/DSS protocol among four different murine strains (BALB/c, C3H/HeN, C57BL/6N, and DBA/2N). The protocol used in this study included a single i.p. injection of AOM (10 mg/kg body weight), followed by 1% DSS in drinking water for 4 days. There was 100% tumor frequency in Balb/c mice and only 50% in C57BL/6N mice. C3H/HeN and DBA/2N mice did not develop adenocarcinomas but only a few adenomas. Interestingly, in mice subjected to AOM injection followed by 0.25% or 0.1% of DSS in drinking water, only dysplastic crypts were observed and no colon tumors were reported.

Histogenesis of Colon Cancer in AOM/DSS Model - from the Emergence of Precancerous Lesions to Late Carcinomas

Colon carcinogenesis, irrespective of animal species, is a focal and sequential process originating from a single colonic crypt. Colon cancer is thought to develop by a multistep process in which normal crypts are initiated to form foci of aberrant crypts (ACF) that proliferate by crypt fission to form microadenoma.

The microadenomas enlarge to give macroscopic adenomas, adenomatous polyps, and finally adenocarcinomas. Thus there is a morphological and genetic progression through an adenoma–carcinoma sequence.

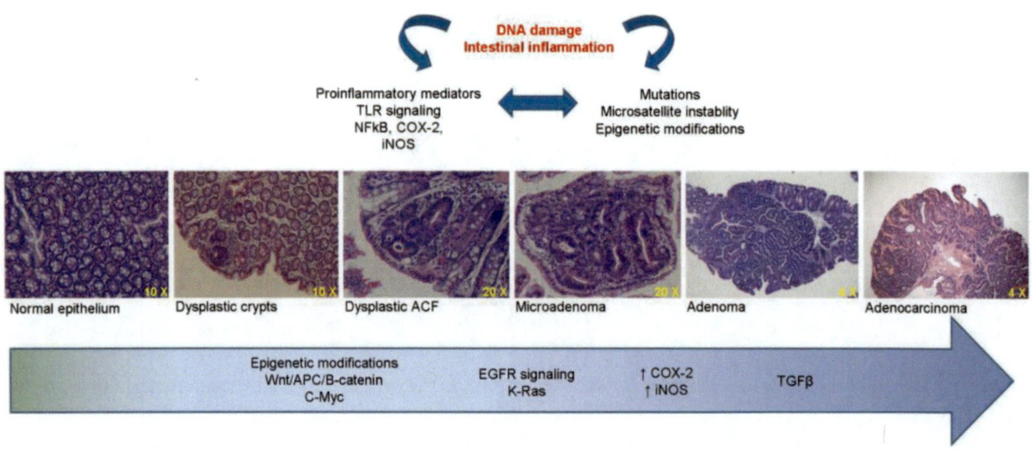

Figure 2. Multistep tumor progression in the AOM/DSS murine model. Hematoxylin-eosin stained colon sections of AOM/DSS treated mice show the ACF-adenoma-carcinoma sequence observed in the model. The principal molecular alterations due to DNA damage induced by AOM, and inflammation stimulus elicited by DSS, are also schematically reported along the multistep tumor progression.

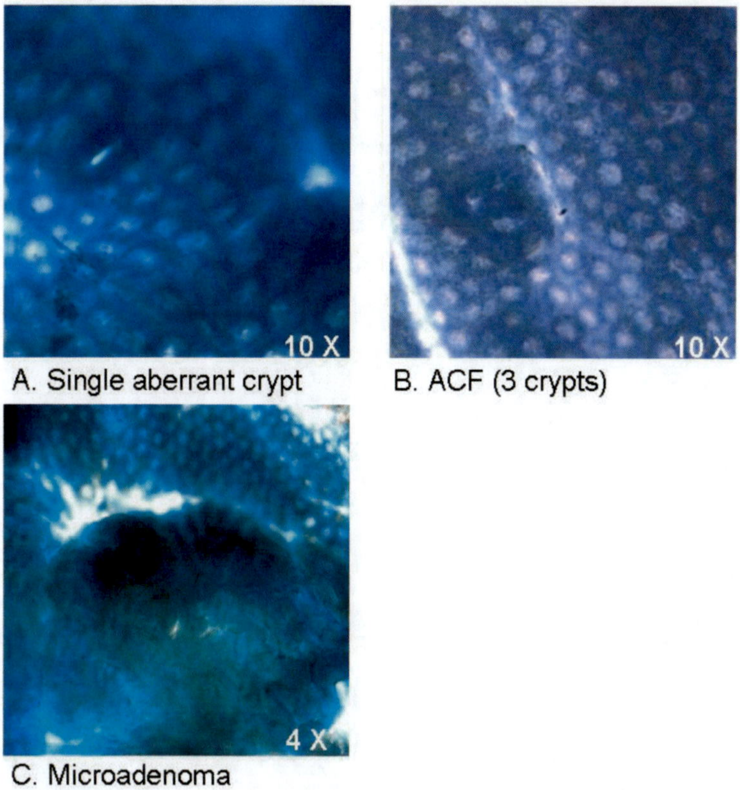

Figure 3. Methylene Blue staining of early colonic lesions developed in mice induced with AOM/DSS treatment. Single aberrant crypt (a); aberrant crypt focus - ACF (b); microadenoma (c). Original magnification, (a, b) ×10; (c) ×4.

The growth, morphological and molecular features of ACF support the definition of ACF as preneoplastic lesions, leading to the extension of the traditional "adenoma-carcinoma" sequence of colorectal carcinogenesis to "ACF-adenoma-carcinoma" sequence. Identification of ACF both in carcinogen-treated rodents and in human colon makes the study of CRC at precancerous stages possible.

Such multistep tumor development can be efficiently reproduced in the AOM/DSS murine model with high reproducibility in both inbred (Balb/c) and outbred [crj:CD-1 (ICR)] susceptible murine strains, as resumed in Figure 2.

Usually, 3–10 macroscopic tumors develop in 80%–100% of the animals, with tubular adenoma, dysplasia, and rarely colitis with mucosal ulceration being present in male mice of susceptible strains at week 10-12 from the start of the treatment.

Colonic crypts can easily be observed by light-microscopic surface examination of formalin-fixed colon preparations stained with methylene blue. When examined in this way, colons of animals that have been treated with AOM/DSS 3–4 weeks earlier are found to have occasional, abnormally large, darkly staining, and slightly raised 'aberrant crypts', as shown in Figure 4. They closely resemble the aberrant crypts seen in patients with both sporadic CRC and FAP.

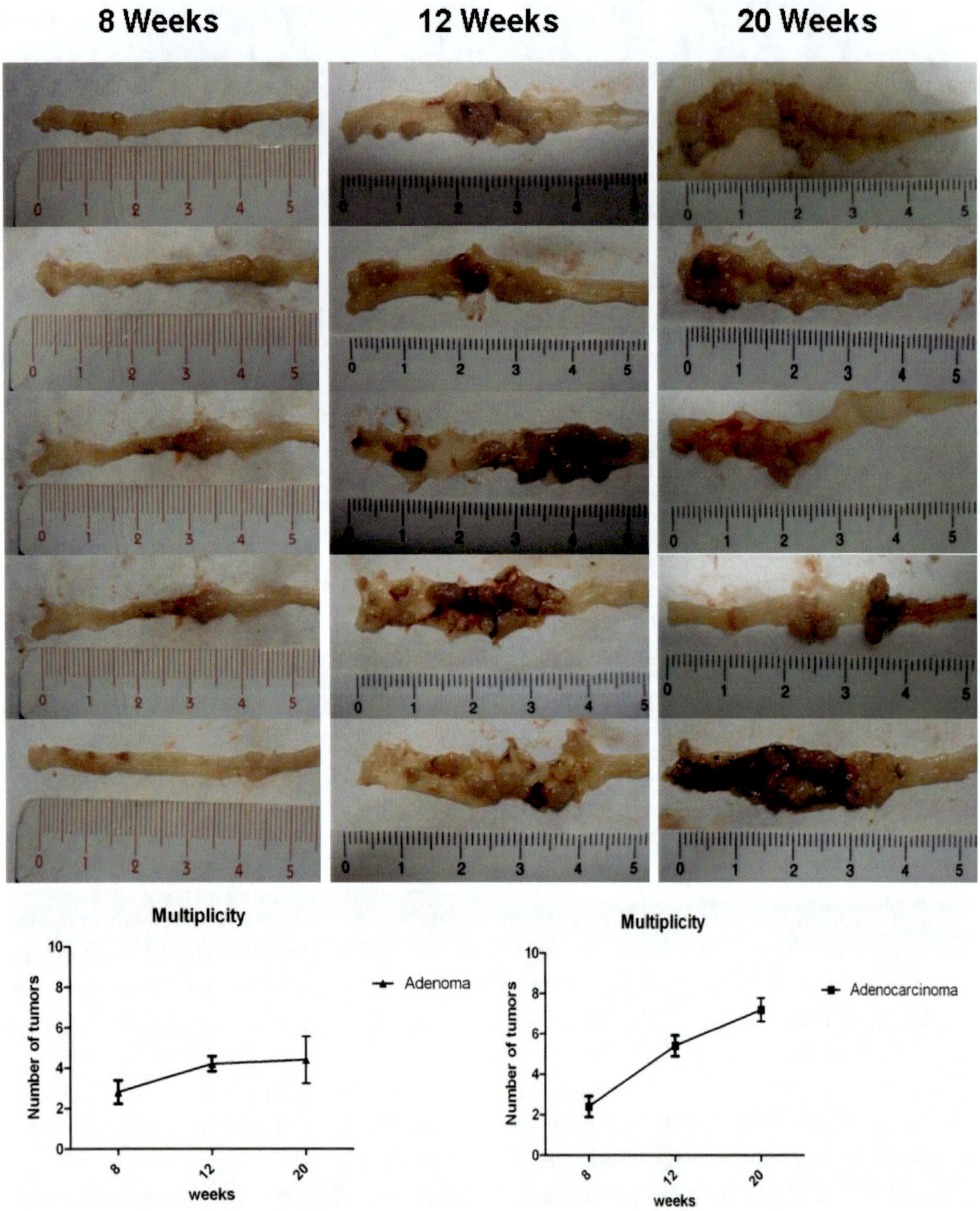

Figure 4. Macroscopic observation showing late colonic neoplasms developed in AOM/DSS-treated mice at 8, 12, and 20 weeks from the start of the AOM/DSS protocol. Tumorsarelocalizedexclusively within thedistal colon. Multiplicity (number of tumors per colon) data are also reported.

In 1987, Bird and Good [52] described ACF as preneoplastic lesions in the colon of carcinogen-treated rodents. Since the total number (crypt multiplicity) and size of these small lesions can be scored easily, ACF have been used as a short-term bioassay to evaluate the role of nutritional components and chemopreventive agents at an early stage of colon carcinogenesis. The aberrant crypts are larger and have a thicker epithelial lining than normal crypts, and are usually gathered together in foci of one to many hundreds of aberrant crypts.

At weeks 3–4 from the start of the AOM/DSS protocol, surface examination of the luminal mucosa of colon preparations reveals flat ACF, classical elevated ACF, and nascent tumors.

Flat ACF have a bright blue appearance and a compressed pit pattern of the crypt openings. Flat ACF and nascent tumors display a uniform picture of severe dysplasia. Apparently, they represent the same type of dysplastic lesions at different stages of crypt multiplication. In contrast, classical elevated ACF do not seem to be as clearly related to tumorigenesis. Furthermore, flat ACF have been shown to grow significantly faster than classical elevated ACF.

Although ACF share many morphological, genetic, and biochemical features with colonic tumors, the association between ACF formation and tumorigenesis is not a simple one. Importantly, in carcinogen-treated rodents, a negative correlation between ACF formation and tumor formation and a discrepancy between distribution of ACF and distribution of tumors has been reported.

Recent findings of the presence of β-catenin accumulated aberrant crypts (BCAC) [53], mucin-depleted crypts (MDF) [54], and flat dysplastic ACF (FDACF) [55] in AOM/DSS-treated rodents are significant advances in the identification of events leading to tumor development. The morphological features of these lesions resemble those of advanced ACF, strongly suggesting that they may be subtypes of advanced ACF. However, the exact evolutionary sequence of BCAC, MDF, or FDACF and their relevance to the human situation is still unclear.

Many aberrant crypts on histological examination show a high level of dysplasia and are then correctly called microadenoma (more than 10 crypts, each less than 1 mm in size) [52]. As microadenomas grow, they might evolve to macroscopic adenoma and, eventually, colon cancer.

AOM/DSS-induced tumors typically display adenomatous growth before showing malignant degeneration and invading the bowel wall, and they are frequently infiltrated by T lymphocytes and other immune cells. On macroscopic examination, nodular, polypoid, or caterpillar-like colonic tumors are exclusively observed in the middle and distal colon of AOM/DSS-treated mice, as in Figure 4. According to Ward, histologically these tumors can be tubular adenoma or well/moderately differentiated tubular adenocarcinoma. [25] The incidences of adenocarcinoma and tubular adenoma at the 20th week is 100% and 38% with a multiplicity of 5.60±2.42 and 0.20±0.40, respectively. Similarly, there is an incidence of 100% of adenomas and 50% of adenocarcinomas as early as week 8, with a multiplicity of 4±1.6 and 0.3±0.7, respectively. After 21 weeks from the start of treatment, only few adenocarcinomas are observed to invade the submucosa, muscularis propria, or serosa [29,30].

Microscopically, these tumors display the characteristics of intraepithelial neoplasia, with changes ranging from low grade dysplasia (usually located at the periphery of polyps, next to non-dysplastic colonic epithelium) to high-grade dysplasia/intramucosal carcinoma (predominantly forming the central parts of the tumors and infiltrating to the submucosa).

Colonic mucosal ulceration with focal dysplasia can be found in the distal colon of mice. Colitis is usually graded on hematoxylin-eosin stained sections as showing a) normal appearance (grade 0); b) mild infiltration of lamina propria by inflammatory cells, with no erosion (grade 1); and c) deep erosion with marked inflammation, often including crypt abscess formation (grade 2) [29]. Mucosal ulceration (grade 2) and colitis with mild erosion can be found in mice at 2 weeks from the end of DSS administration, but the inflammatory state progressively decreases in the following weeks and a resolution of the acute inflammation can be observed at weeks 5-6 [30].

Molecular Events Associated with Colon Carcinogenesis in the AOM/DSS Model and Relevance for Human CRC

The transition from normal epithelium through adenoma to carcinoma is associated with the acquisition of molecular events. Among the earliest events in the human colorectal tumor progression pathway is the loss of function of the APC gene product, which appears to be consistent with its important role in predisposing persons with germline APC mutations to colorectal tumors. Acquired or inherited mutations of DNA damage-repair genes also play a role in predisposing colorectal epithelial cells to mutations.

Studies in mice and rats have revealed that AOM/DSS induced tumors display very similar features to human CRC even at the molecular level. In a recent study, a comprehensive protein expression analysis in the AOM/DSS model revealed an aberrant expression of proteins functionally related to metabolism, antioxidant system, oxidative stress, mucin production, and inflammation [56].

Moreover, this protocol could provide a powerful murine model to mechanistically investigate CIN (chromosomal instability) in colitis-associated carcinogenesis. Remarkably, despite CRCs induced by administration of AOM alone, which therefore arise devoid of chronic inflammation, are genetically stable, it has been reported that a high percentage of tumors that arise after AOM/DSS treatment exhibit CIN (81.25%) [57].

Consistent with findings in human CRC, AOM/DSS-induced tumors have mutations of APC, K-Ras and increased levels of enzymes involved in prostaglandin and nitric oxide synthesis, such as cyclooxygenase-2 (COX-2) and inducible nitric oxide synthase (iNOS), but no immunoreactivity to p53.

Wnt/APC/β-Catenin Pathway

Tumors in the AOM/DSS model, similarly to the *ApcMin/+* mice, have signaling alterations marked by the aberrantly activated canonical Wnt pathway, which is normally involved in repressing differentiation during embryogenesis and in the postembryonic regulation of cell positioning in the intestinal crypts.

Inactivating APC mutations or activating β-catenin mutations, which mimic Wnt stimulation and lead to β-catenin accumulation, are reported to be early events of colorectal carcinogenesis in both humans and rodents [58].

In contrast to human colon cancers, where the β-catenin gene is frequently mutated at codons 33, 41, and 45 of the glycogen synthase kinase-3β (GSK-3β) phosphorylation motif, mutations in AOM/DSS-induced CRC are found at codons 32, 33, and 34. This location is slightly different from that mentioned in another report, where β-catenin gene mutations of murine tumors induced by AOM are present at codons 33, 34, 37, and 41, but not at codon 32 [58]. It has been reported that the β-catenin mutations at codons 37 and 41, which are important serine and threonine sites for GSK-3β phosphorylation, possess high oncogenic potential.

Since β-catenin gene mutations have been detected at codon 32, 34, 37, and 41 in DMH/DSS-induced colon adenocarcinoma [59], the different mutational spectra observed in the β-catenin gene directly relates to the particular carcinogenic treatment given. Therefore, it has been speculated that DSS exposure causes a shift in the mutation sites from that induced by treatment with DMH or AOM alone. A large upregulation of the T-cell factor-4 (Tcf-4) transcript can be also observed in AOM/DSS-induced tumors [60].

K-Ras

As in human CRC, K-Ras mutations are involved in the early stages of AOM/DSS colorectal carcinogenesis and are associated with increased tumor size. The mutated forms of Ras are found to stimulate cell proliferation, transformation, and differentiation. Consistent with findings in human CRC, K-Ras activation appears to play an important role both in the AOM and the DMH models, whereas this pathway is not frequently targeted by PhIP. It has been shown that DMH caused K-Ras-activating mutations (G to A) in 66% of colon mouse carcinomas [61].

c-Myc

c-Myc works as a global mediator of the oncogenic process and is often increased in human CRC. The gene is a direct transcriptional target of the Wnt/β-catenin pathway, while the transforming growth factor-β (TGF-β) signaling is associated with c-Myc repression through SMAD3, binding to a repressive SMAD-binding element (RSBE) within the c-Myc promoter. Mouse models have been used to show that decreased c-Myc expression leads to reduced numbers of CRCs, [62] a result confirmed by c-Myc inhibition in human CRC. Recently, an increased expression of c-Myc and telomerase (TERT) has been observed in foci of high-grade dysplasia/intramucosal carcinoma isolated from AOM/DSS-treated Crj:CD-1 (ICR) mice [63,60]. Of note, telomerase not only compensates for natural telomere erosion and thus contributes to permanent cell growth, but it is also able to activate progenitor cells by controlling c-Myc- and Wnt-related transcription pathways [64].

TGF-β

Sporadic CRCs often acquire resistance to TGF-β signaling. At later stages of cancer progression there is increased expression of TGF-β, promoting invasion and metastasis.

It has been shown that in TGF-β receptor-deficient and TGF-β transgenic mice after treatment with AOM there is a significantly greater development of tumors than in wild-type mice [65].

Particularly, only TGF-β1 protein is upregulated in the colonic mucosa of mice treated with AOM/DSS, whereas TGF-β3 is a notable downregulated gene [63].

Cox-2

The COX-2 protein is found in the cytoplasm of neoplastic colonic epithelial cells and to a lesser extent in stromal cells, whereas normal epithelium is negative for COX-2. It is a cytoplasmic protein that catalyzes the synthesis of lipid inflammatory mediators (prostaglandins and prostacyclins) from arachidonic acid. Expression is increased at sites of inflammation as well as in ~80% of CRCs and 40% of colorectal adenomas.

AOM augments the expression of cyclooxygenase (COX)-2 (but not COX-1) in colonic tumors [66], which, in turn, suppresses TGFBR2 expression [67] and activates intrinsic tyrosine kinase of epidermal growth factor receptor (EGFR) [68] in laboratory rodents.

After AOM/DSS challenge, the expression of COX-2 is upregulated in neoplastic cells in mice with mutations in the tumor suppressor Apc [69]. COX-2 may contribute to tumor development by modulating apoptosis, angiogenesis, and tumor invasiveness. It also has a role in the progression of cancer via activation of metalloproteases, thereby increasing the invasiveness of colon cancer cells.

iNOS

All tumors as well as dysplasias that develop in the AOM/DSS model show positive reactivity for iNOS [29]. Such enzyme catalyzes the production of nitric oxide from L-arginine and is an important cellular signaling molecule, playing a vital role as intercellular signal generator in the control of vascular tone, insulin secretion, and airway tone.

A lack of correlation between immunohistochemical signal/Western blot assay and iNOS mRNA levels found in tumors of AOM/DSS model [29,70], should be explained by iNOS extracellular localization. iNOS overexpression is indeed partly localized to tumor stroma, especially to tumor-associated macrophages. It is also possible that there is no simple relationship between steady-state transcript level and mature protein. Finally, it has been speculated that mouse iNOS is not essential for the development of colitis-associated tumorigenesis [71], even though iNOS inhibition attenuates tumorigenesis in mice treated with DSS [72].

p53 Pathway

The ARF/p53 pathway, which is effective at limiting the proliferation and survival of oncogenically transformed cells, appears to be dysregulated during the carcinogenic process in humans. However, p53 immunohistochemical expression has not been detected in AOM/DSS-induced colonic dysplasia and neoplasms [29].

Immunohistochemical observation revealed that only a few colonic tumors induced by DSS show positive reactivity against p53 [73], and both ARF and p53sequences are normal in

AOM-induced colon tumors but, strikingly, the ability of p53 to activate or repress transcription is suppressed [74].

This observation may induce to assume that non genetic inhibition of p53 may play a critical role in colon carcinogenesis in the absence of p53 sequence alterations, suggesting a role for posttranslational modifications in suppressing p53 activity in AOM-induced tumors.

Epigenetic Modifications

Recent studies have suggested that alterations in DNA methylation can contribute to tumor pathogenesis in mouse models similarly to what happens in human cancer. A global DNA hypomethylation is indeed observed in human colorectal malignancy as well as in tumors arising in the AOM-induced mouse model [75], although the frequency of aberrantly methylated genes in such mouse model appears to be less common than in human CRC.

The methylation status of normal, inflamed, and dysplastic colonic tissue has been studied intensively. It has been proposed that gene methylation may be an early event in inflammation-associated tumorigenesis, and thus can potentially be a sensitive marker for predicting dysplasia.

Recently, the AOM colon cancer model has been used for assessing the methylation state of tumor suppressor genes to determine the role of epigenetic alterations in cancer initiation and progression.

Among a number of candidate genes known to be aberrantly methylated in human cancer or mouse tumor models, two genes, Zik1 (zinc finger protein-interacting with K protein 1) and Gja9 (gap junction protein alpha-9), undergo aberrant DNA methylation in AOM-induced tumors, which is either not present or is present at low frequency in the normal colon [76]. The aberrant DNA methylation of Gja9 has not been reported previously, instead the hypermethylation of Zik1 has also been identified in intestinal metaplasia (IM) of the stomach, in gastric cancer cell lines, and in primary gastric cancer tumor samples, suggesting that epigenetic silencing of Zik1 may contribute to the pathogenesis of gastric neoplasia and may play an important role in the transformation of gastrointestinal mucosa from normal to cancerous.

Early studies of the epigenetic modifications occurring in the AOM-based CRC murine models indicate that AOM-induced mouse colonic tumors can also recapitulate the epigenetic aberrations of human CRC. However, further analysis using genome-wide approaches should provide a comprehensive assessment of the methylation state of the DNA in colon cancers arising in AOM murine models in order to highlight the potential of these models to study a range of issues that remains to be resolved in the field of human epigenetic aberrations.

Pathogenesis and Molecular Biology of Colitis-Induced Carcinogenesis in the AOM/DSS Model

A role for inflammation in tumorigenesis is now generally accepted, and it has become evident that an inflammatory microenvironment is an essential component of all tumors, including some in which a direct causal relationship with inflammation is not yet proven.

Accumulated evidences, obtained using *in vivo* and *in vitro* disease models and the analysis of clinical patient samples, strongly favors the theory that both precancerous inflammation and inflammation stemming from genetic alterations can cause cell transformation and promote tumor progression. The roles and the relationship between the two pathways in the cancer development process depend on their specific interactions between genetic/epigenetic factors and environmental factors.

Epidemiological studies have attributed up to 25% of cancer deaths worldwide to chronic inflammation, which is generally caused by genetic mutations, autoimmune diseases, and exposure to environmental factors. Among chronic inflammation associated with microbial infections, the bacterium *Helicobacter pylori*, is one of the main contributing factors to the development of gastric cancer, the second most common cause of cancer-related mortality worldwide. Furthermore, *Helicobacter hepaticus* infection accelerates AOM-induced tumorigenesis compared to AOM treatment alone in IL-10 knocked-out mice, that promotes inflammation mediated colonic tumor growth [77].

Interestingly, tumors of the gastrointestinal tract provide a paradigmatic connection between inflammation and cancer. Epidemiological studies have shown that patients with IBD, including UC, are at increased risk of developing CRC. IBD-associated colon carcinogenesis can be summarized as an inflammation–dysplasia–carcinoma sequence: hyperplastic lesions in the inflamed mucosa develop CRC after passing through the phase of flat dysplasia.

A number of possible mechanisms by which inflammation can contribute to carcinogenesis have been elucidated, including induction of genomic instability, alterations in epigenetic events and subsequent aberrant gene expression. The cancer stem cell model postulates that expansion of stem cells occurs in response to these mutations, resulting in tumor formation. Multiple pathways are likely to play a role, including production of reactive oxygen species and cytokine and chemokine expression by immune cells, which increase the risk of mutagenesis, and interactions between cancer stem cells and the local tumor microenvironment, including immune cells and myofibroblasts. Inflammation also affects DNA methylation patterns and histone modifications.

The AOM/DSS model represents a highly reliable tool to examine the role of inflammation as a driving force in colon carcinogenesis. It is very useful compared to a standard UC model, which typically requires long exposure periods or many cycles of DSS administration, before resulting in a relatively low tumor incidence [78].

At 3–4 weeks from AOM/DSS treatment, the colonic mucosa of AOM/DSS-treated mice displays signs of diffuse colitis and high numbers of inflammatory cells are contained in the lamina propria. Although the inflammatory stimulus acts as the principal driving force for the initial tumor development promotion, after 5-6 weeks from the start of the protocol the colitis tissue injury appears completely repaired, while carcinogenesis progression is advancing. Interestingly, extensive mast cell migration can be found surrounding or within carcinomas [29]. This parallels what is observed in humans, where colitis-associated cancer is characterized by a dense infiltrate of immune cells.

During the initiation and promotion phase of tumor development in the AOM/DSS model both conditions predisposing to cancer can be observed: colitis and genetic/epigenetic events. Such conditions are fundamental to coordinate a particular microenvironment which contributes to tumor progression.

Key components of cancer-promoting inflammation have been investigated in the AOM/DSS model.

Proinflammatory Factors

NFkB - The NFkB signaling pathway is a key coordinator of innate immunity and inflammation. It plays crucial roles in both precancerous chronic inflammation as well as cancer induced inflammation. Frequently activated by cancer gene mutation, TLRs (Toll-like receptors), or by TNF-α and IL-1β, NFkB is an important regulator of tumor initiation and progression. Activation of this pathway induces expression of inflammatory cytokines, adhesion molecules, enzymes in the prostaglandin-synthesis pathway (such as COX2), iNOS, angiogenic factors and anti-apoptotic genes (such as Bcl-2).

When NFkB activity is disrupted in colonic epithelial cells of AOM/DSS-treated mice, there is a dramatic reduction in tumor number [79]. This is associated with enhanced epithelial cell apoptosis during early tumor development, but there is no reduction in inflammation.

The overexpression of netrin-1, a transcriptional target for NFkB, in AOM/DSS-treated mice parallels a similar alteration in CRCs from IBD patients [80].

TNF-α - TNF-α is a key regulator of inflammation, inducing the recruitment of intracellular adaptor proteins. Its receptor (TNFR) can trigger NFkB and downstream cell survival pathways as well as caspase-8 and associated apoptotic pathways. In CRC, the protein levels of TNF-α are abnormally increased in the preneoplastic inflamed colonic mucosa [81]. TNFR1 knockout mice showed a much milder form of colitis with a reduced tumor incidence in response to the AOM/DSS treatment as compared to wild-type mice [82]. Furthermore, the specific TNF-α antagonist etanercept not only suppresses colitis in AOM/DSS treated mice but also efficiently prevents the tumor formation [81].

IL-6 - Among the proinflammatory cytokines, interestingly IL-6 signaling inhibition reduces tumor development in AOM-induced model, suggesting IL-6 trans-signaling plays a pivotal role in the development of colon cancer [83]. IL-6 expressed during colitis is shown to promote tumor growth in mice. In this model, selective inhibition of the TGFβ signaling in T cells is associated with an enhanced expression of IL-6.

IL-21 - Interleukin-21 is a key regulator of the proliferation and/or effector function of B cells, T cells, and natural killer cells, and also affects regulatory T cells. It has been shown that IL-21 is overexpressed in the colonic mucosa of UC patients, where it positively regulates Th17 cell responses. Similarly, IL-21 knockout mice that underwent AOM/DSS treatment, show reduced mucosal damage, reduced infiltration of T cells, and diminished production of IL-6 and IL-17A. IL-21–deficient mice also develop fewer and smaller tumors compared with wild-type mice [84].

Regulatory Factors

TGFβ - Similar to NFkB, the STAT3-TGFβ signaling pathway is involved in numerous oncogenic signaling pathways. These transcription factors are constitutively activated in tumor cells and are involved in oncogenesis and inhibition of apoptosis. The activation of

STAT3 in tumor cells has also been implicated in immune evasion via inhibition of dendritic cell maturation and the subsequent immune response.

In the AOM/DSS model, an increased activation of STAT1 and STAT3 is observed because of a loss of Socs1 and Socs3 (suppressors of cytokine signaling) expression [85].

AOM/DSS-induced adenocarcinomas from Socs1-deficient mice have increased levels of nuclear β-catenin and Myc expression when compared to tumors of wild-type mice, showing a direct link between Socs signaling and Myc [85]. The deficiency of Socs3 in the intestine does not lead to chronic inflammation or development of tumors in mice. However, when treated with AOM/DSS, these mice develop colon tumors that are preceded by inflammation, suggesting that Socs3 expression in the neighboring stroma may be required to suppress chronic inflammation and, subsequently, tumor promotion.

IL-10 - Interleukin-10 is a key anti-inflammatory cytokine produced primarily by monocytes, T cells and B cells. IL-10 can block NFkB activity, and also regulates the JAK Stat signaling pathway. It is also known as human cytokine synthesis inhibitory factor (CSIF).

IL-10 knockout mice develop spontaneous colitis-associated cancer, which is associated with the overproduction of Th1 cytokine. The AOM/DSS protocol promotes inflammation-mediated colonic tumor growth in IL-10 knockout mice [57].

Chemokines

Chemokines and their receptors play an integral role in IBD by regulating the accumulation of immune cells at the site of intestinal inflammation. In the AOM/DSS model, mice deficient for D6, a promiscuous decoy receptor that scavenges several inflammatory chemokines, show increased expression of chemokines and higher accumulation of inflammatory cells in comparison to the wild-type, resulting in the development of more severe colitis and higher incidence of tumors [86].

Toll Like Receptors

Of no less importance are the mediators that keep inflammation in check, including toll-like receptors (TLRs).

TLRs play a major role in sensing gut microbiota and activation of these receptors is required to maintain intestinal homeostasis. Genetic or functional disregulation of TLRs may be linked to chronic inflammation and tumor development.

TLR-4, which responds specifically to bacterial lipopolysaccharide ligand and is expressed at low levels in normal intestinal mucosa, has been shown to be upregulated in the mucosa of patients with IBD, in UC-associated CRC, and in colon tumors that develop in the AOM/DSS mouse model [87]. TLR4 may lower the threshold for carcinogenesis in the AOM/DSS-induced cancer model [88]. In the same model, endogenous administration of prostaglandin E2 (PGE2) treatment increases mucosal expression of COX-2, suggesting that PGE2 is involved in the TLR-4-mediated intestinal tumorigenesis [89].

Recently it has been shown that MyD88, the TLR adaptor protein, plays a protective role in the development of the AOM/DSS colitis-associated cancer, due in part to the IL-18 receptor signal activation [90].

TIR8

TIR8, the single immunoglobulin IL-1 receptor-related molecule (SIGIRR), a negative regulator for Toll-IL-1R signaling, plays a critical role in gut homeostasis, intestinal inflammation, and colitis-associated tumorigenesis by maintaining the microbial tolerance of the colonic epithelium. In the AOM/DSS mouse model, TIR8-/- mice show a strong increase in inflammation related cancer susceptibility in comparison to wild-type mice [91].

These results unequivocally demonstrate the important role of inflammation in CRC progression.

Heparanase

Heparanase is causally involved in inflammation and accelerates colon tumorigenesis associated with IBD. It is constantly overexpressed by the colonic epithelium in human UC as well as in the AOM/DSS murine model, where its overexpression preserves a chronic inflammatory conditions in DSS colitis and thus creates a tumor promoting microenvironment characterized by enhanced NFkB signaling, STAT3 induction, and increased vascularization [36].

Oxidative Stress and DNA Damage

Inflammatory cells produce a variety of reactive oxygen and nitrogen species which may generate gene mutations and DNA damage, leading to carcinogenesis.

Direct genotoxicity has been documented in mouse models of intestinal inflammation, which correlates with the degree of systemic and local inflammation, and has been associated with evidence of reactive oxygen species-mediated oxidative stress and DNA damage. The AOM/DSS model contributed to demonstrate that mice which are deficient in base excision repair enzymes have increased tumor multiplicity after AOM/DSS treatment, confirming that inflammation can induce DNA damage which in turn contributes to colon carcinogenesis [92,50].

The AOM/DSS Model in Preclinical Studies

Despite surveillance colonoscopy or prophylactic colectomy, the concept of chemoprevention has gained increasing importance during the last years. Many pharmacological agents have been evaluated for their chemopreventive features for inflammation-associated CRC. To this purpose, several natural and synthetic compounds have been assayed using the AOM/DSS induced mouse colorectal carcinogenesis model, which can be considered a valuable *in vivo* platform for chemopreventive intervention studies.

All these compounds have anti-inflammatory activity and are able to suppress the expression of COX-2, iNOS, and inflammatory cytokines. Several are promising preventive or therapeutical compounds and their clinical application is expected.

Natural Plant Compounds

Lots of representative chemopreventive compounds belong to the class of natural plant compounds.

Epidemiological studies clearly demonstrate the existence of an inverse correlation between a diet rich in fruits/vegetables and human colon cancer. Fruits and vegetables contain indeed active compounds able to reduce the risk of this tumor.

- *Prenyloxycoumarins*, including auraptene and collinin, from citrus fruits, are reported to have anti-inflammatory activity. The effects of these natural compounds have been examined in AOM/DSS mouse colon carcinogenesis model, since dietary administration of auraptene and collinin could effectively suppress colitis-related colon carcinogenesis induced by AOM and DSS [72]. The incidence of colorectal adenocarcinomas in AOM/DSS mouse with different dosages (0.01% and 0.05%) of auraptene and collinin is significantly lower than that in the untreated mice. The multiplicity of colon adenocarcinomas and colonic inflammation scores in those mice is also significantly lower than that of the controls. The suppressive effect of auraptene and collinin on the development of colonic adenocarcinoma correlates with the inhibition of cell proliferation activity, induction of apoptosis, and inhibition of immunoreactivity of COX-2 and iNOS in the colonic malignancies. Thus the protective effects of dietary prenyloxycoumarins after treatment with AOM and DSS might be mainly due to their ability to inhibit inflammation and oxidative stress.

Furthermore, the chemopreventive property of auraptene and a novel prodrug, 4'-geranyloxy-ferulic acid (GOFA), has been tested using inclusion complexes with beta-cyclodextrin (β-CD):GOFA/β-CD and AUR/β-CD. These compounds exert their chemopreventive effect by modulating cell proliferation, inducing apoptosis, and suppressing proinflammatory cytokines in adenocarcinomas that develop in the setting of colitis. It has been demonstrated that treatment with GOFA/β-CD and AUR/β-CD significantly lowers colonic inflammation induced by DSS in the AOM/DSS model [93].

- Herbal medicines, such as *ginseng*, are able to potentiate the effects of chemotherapeutic agents via synergistic activities, as antioxidant, anti-proliferative and anti-inflammatory effects. Ginseng consists of over 100 ginsenosides as the major biologically active constituents, in addition to many peptides and poly saccharides. It has been shown that American Ginseng (AG), a putative non-toxic antioxidant can both prevent and treat AOM/DSS-induced colitis-driven colon cancer. In this model, it has been demonstrated that ginseng could suppress EGFR signals in colonic tumorigenesis [94].

Another recent study, using AOM/DSS treated mice fed Western diet (containing 20% fat), has revealed that oral ginseng ingestion inhibits drug induced colitis and colonic tumorigenesis. It appears that Compound K (the final metabolite of ginsenoside Rb1) plays an important role in the observed effects [95].

- Other essential antioxidant nutrients, *tocopherols and tocotrienols*, collectively known as vitamin E, have been recently analyzed in mouse and human samples. In this context, the AOM/DSS model contributed to assess the first comprehensive simultaneous analysis of different side-chain metabolites of tocopherols and tocotrienols in mice and humans, demonstrating that urinary metabolites may serve as useful biomarkers for nutritional assessment of vitamin E [96].
- *Resveratrol* is a naturally occurring polyphenol. It is recognized as one of the more promising natural molecules in the prevention and treatment of chronic inflammatory and autoimmune disorders, and exhibits cardio- and cancer-protective activities.

Resveratrol has been tested in the AOM/DSS model and a significant reduction of tumor incidence and multiplicity was observed in mice treated compared to the controls. The study indicated that resveratrol is a useful, non-toxic complementary and alternative strategy to abate colitis and potentially colon cancer associated with colitis [97].

In a previous study, it was reported that 2,3′,4,4′,5′-pentamethoxy-*trans*-stilbene (PMS), a methoxylated resveratrol derivative, exerts a highly potent anti-proliferative effect on human colon cancer cells as compared with its parent compound. Subsequently, the chemopreventive effect of PMS has been evaluated in the AOM/DSS model. Intragastric administration of PMS (25, 50 mg/kg body weight) for 16 weeks significantly reduced the multiplicity of colonic neoplasms by 15% and 35% ($P < 0.01$) respectively. Moreover, PMS at 50 mg/kg inhibited colon cancer cell proliferation and promoted apoptosis. Such changes are accompanied by reduction of Akt (protein kinase B) phosphorylation, inactivation of β-catenin and down-regulation of iNOS [98].

- Recent works have elucidated several biological properties of *zerumbone* (ZER), a major constituent of the subtropical ginger plant, which seems to inhibit carcinogenesis through inhibition of free radical generation, iNOS and COX-2 expression, and TNF-α release in activated leukocytes, as well as induction of apoptosis in human colonic adenocarcinoma cell lines.

Dietary feeding with ZER strongly suppresses DSS-induced acute colitis in mice [99] and the formation of aberrant crypt foci (ACF). It also reduces the incidence and the multiplicity of colonic adenocarcinoma in mice receiving ZER at different doses (100 ppm, 250 ppm, and 500 ppm). ZER feeding significantly decreases the PCNA labeling index and lowers the immunohistochemical scores of NFkB and HO-1 (heme oxygenase), the expression of which correlates with carcinogenesis and inflammation.

- *Silibinin*, a flavonolignan isolated from *Silybum marianum*, has been tested in the AOM mouse model. Interestingly, both low (250 mg/kg) and high (750 mg/kg) doses of silibinin, besides inhibiting cell proliferation and inducing apoptosis, impacts the levels of inflammatory and angiogenic mediators such as COX-2, iNOS, and VEGF, suggesting that silibinin has chemopreventive efficacy in colon tumorigenesis due to its effects on two key events of colon carcinogenesis: inflammation and angiogenesis [100].

- *Phenethyl isothiocyanate (PEITC) and dibenzoylmethane (DBM)*, both metabolites of vegetable compounds, are potent natural dietary compounds for chemoprevention of colon cancer induced by AOM/DSS and appear to be associated with different *in vivo* mechanism of actions. PEITC's chemopreventive effect seems to be due to induction of apoptosis and cell cycle arrest, whereas DBM's effect is due to prevention of AOM initiation via induction of Nrf2 and phase II detoxifying enzymes [101].
- *Tricin*, the flavone 4',5,7-trihydroxy-3',5-dimethoxyflavone present in rice, oats, barley, and wheat exhibits antigrowth activity in several human cancer cell lines and anti-inflammatory potential. The chemopreventive activity has been elucidated for the first time in male Crj: CD-1 mice subjected to AOM/DSS treatment [102].

  This study has demonstrated that dietary tricin, containing 50 or 250 ppm dose of tricin, inhibits inflammation-related mouse colon carcinogenesis by suppressing the expression of TNF-α in the nonlesional cyrpts and the proliferation of adenocarcinomas. A potential use of tricin for clinical trials of colorectal cancer chemoprevention has been suggested.

Modulation of Physiological Molecules

The AOM/DSS model has also been used to investigate the role of physiological molecule as remedy for colitis associated carcinogenesis.

- The effects of *selenium(Se)* have been studied in colon carcinogenesis, because of the ability of supplemental Se to reduce the incidence and mortality of colon cancer in humans. Also, several animal studies have shown the protective effects of Se against aberrant crypt formation and colon tumor development [103,104]. The effects of Se in colon carcinogenesis have been recently studied with the administration of three different levels of Se and high-iron diet to the AOM/DSS mouse model, to investigate the relationship between the iron and the risk of colorectal cancer. Experimental results suggested that dietary Se supplement may have protective effect against colon cancer by decreasing proliferation, increasing apoptosis of tumor cells, and reducing oxidative stress in mice with high iron diet [105].

These data are confirmed by a recent study, combining in mice the AOM/DSS treatment with feeding wild-type and GPx2 (gastrointestinal glutathione peroxidase) knockout mice a moderately Se-deficient, Se-adequate, and Se-supranutritional diet [106].

- Moreover, *8-hydroxydeoxyguanosine (8-OHdG)*, widely used in many studies as a biomarker for the measurement of endogenous oxidative DNA damage, and as a risk factor for many diseases including cancer, has been investigated in the AOM/DSS model to determine whether exogenous 8-OHdG has a preventive effect on colitis and colitis-associated cancer [107]. Daily injections of 8-OHdG significantly inhibit recruitment of inflammatory cells in DSS-induced colitis. Additionally, a chronic ingestion of diet containing 8-OHdG exerts a chemopreventive role in AOM/DSS-induced colitis associated cancer [108].

- In the last years, it has been reported that the membrane-associated mammalian sialidase *NEU3*, which preferentially acts on gangliosides, is involved in cell differentiation, motility, and tumorigenesis. The NEU3 gene expression is aberrantly elevated in several human cancers, including colon, renal, prostate, and ovarian cancers. In the AOM/DSS model of colon carcinogenesis, no differences in the incidence or growth of tumors between the Neu3-deficient and wild-type mice has been observed. On the other hand, the Neu3-deficient mice are less susceptible than wild-type mice to the colitis-associated colon carcinogenesis induced by AOM/DSS. These results suggest that NEU3 plays an important role in inflammation-dependent tumor development [109].
- Among cytokines, particular attention has recently been paid to *interleukin-21 (IL-21)*, since it seems to play a decisive role in controlling tumorigenesis. Data emerging from pre-clinical and clinical studies indicates that forced overexpression of IL-21 in tumor cells suppresses their growth, through enhanced antitumor immunity. Nonetheless, studies in the AOM/DSS model have strongly supported the tumor-promoting role of IL-21, raising the possibility that IL-21 could have opposing functions on the growth of tumors [84,110].
- Recently, the AOM/DSS model has been used to investigate the role of the *Peroxisome proliferator-activated receptor-γ coactivator 1-α (PGC1α)*, a transcriptional coactivator that interacts with PPARs, which is able to drive mitochondrial biogenesis and respiration in the presence of reduced antioxidant enzyme activities, thus determining the accumulation of reactive oxygen species and fostering the fate of enterocytes toward apoptosis. Such interesting study presented an intriguing scenario whereby PGC1α regulates enterocyte cell fate and protects against tumorigenesis [111].

Synthetic Drugs

PPAR inhibitors - In several studies conducted by Tanaka *et al.*, the chemopreventive ability of different synthetic PPAR ligands was characterized in the AOM/DSS-induced mouse colon carcinogenesis model [112].

Peroxisome proliferator-activated receptors (PPARs) are members of the nuclear hormone receptor superfamily and have been implicated in a variety of physiological and pathological processes, such as nutrient metabolism, energy homeostasis, inflammation and cancer.

Three PPAR isotypes, PPARα, PPARβ, and PPARγ, have been identified. PPARγ is highly expressed in fat tissue and plays an important role in adipocyte differentiation and lipid storage. It is also expressed in a number of epithelial neoplasms, such as cancers in colon, breast, and prostate. PPARγ ligands, such as troglitazone and rosiglitazone can induce apoptosis and adipogenic differentiation and inhibit tumor growth both *in vitro* and *in vivo* [113,114].

Inhibition of inflammation in colon mucosa and decrease in cell proliferation activity caused by these PPAR ligands might be responsible for their chemopreventive effects in the AOM/DSS induced carcinogenesis [115]. A new third-generation thiazolidinedione, RS5444, which is about 50 times more potent than rosiglitazone, has been tested in the AOM/DSS mouse model [116,117].

RS5444 is able to significantly suppress ACF formation in AOM-treated mice and may therefore have chemopreventive efficacy. Moreover, RS5444-treated mice show a decrease of about 30% in tumor incidence, though this reduction is not statistically significant.

Although RS5444 does not inhibit the growth of established tumors, it has been observed that control tumors are significantly more dysplastic than those from RS5444-treated mice.

It seems indeed that PPARγ ligands promote differentiation of both normal and transformed gastrointestinal epithelial cells, consistently with their ability to promote differentiation of minimally transformed colonic epithelial cells. The aptitude to block initiation of transformation may also be explained by their ability to inhibit the proliferation of normal colonic cells, thereby decreasing the numbers of target cells where the carcinogen could act.

SK1 inhibitors - Inhibition of sphingosine kinase 1 (SK1) using either pharmacological inhibitors or by crossing SK1 null mice has shown promise in many xenograft models of cancer as well as several genetic and chemically induced mouse models of carcinogenesis. The evidence suggests that tissue expression of SK1 correlates with cancer stage, chemotherapy response, and tumor aggressiveness.

Since SK inhibitors exert suppression of colitis, a novel SK inhibitor, ABC294640, has been evaluated in the AOM/DSS model. A treatment with this SK inhibitor resulted in a dose-dependent decrease in tumor incidence and multiplicity.

Importantly, with ABC294640, there are no observed toxic side effects. Results of this recent study are consistent with the hypothesis that the inhibition of SK activity by the novel SK inhibitor modulates key pathways involved in cell survival and may be a viable treatment strategy for the chemoprevention of colitis-driven colon cancer [118].

COX-2 inhibitors -Mesalazine or 5-aminosalicylic acid (5-ASA) is a drug widely used in IBDs, and recent observations indicate that mesalazine can be also chemopreventive for IBD-associated CRC, even though the effect of the anti-inflammatory 5-ASA on the risk for colitis-associated CRC is still controversial.

Most of the anti-neoplastic properties of 5-ASA have been attributed to its ability to target mucosal immune cells and inhibit expression and/or activity of various molecules involved in colon carcinogenesis (e.g., COX-2, iNOS, reactive oxygen species and NFkB).

However, mesalazine could also regulate directly the activity of neoplastic cells in a COX-2 independent way.

The effect of 5-ASA and its derivates on colorectal carcinogenesis has been evaluated in the AOM/DSS mouse model where a reduction of number and size of neoplasms has been observed [119].

A study conducted by Clapper *et al.* [120] evaluated the ability of 5-ASA to inhibit colitis-associated colorectal neoplasia in the AOM/DSS model. The results strongly suggest that chronic exposure to 5-ASA is able to reduce susceptibility to colitis-associated CRC.

Table 2. Chemopreventive preclinical trials performed in the AOM/DSS model

Compound	Model and strain	Experimental protocol	Observations	References
Natural plant compounds				
Auraptene / Collinin	1 i.p. AOM (10 mg/kg bw) + 1% DSS in drinking water for 1 wk, 1 wk after AOM. Strain: Male Crj: CD-1 (ICR) mice.	Diet containing auraptene or collinin for 17 wks: 1 wk after the stop of DSS.	Tumor inhibitory effect on colonic adenocarcinoma.	[67]
4'-geranyloxy-ferulic acid (GOFA) and auraptene (AUR)	1 i.p. AOM (10 mg/kg bw) + 1.5% DSS in drinking water for 1 wk, 1 wk after AOM. Strain: Male Crj: CD-1 (ICR) mice.	Basal diet containing 2 dose levels (100 and 500 ppm) of GOFA/β-CD or AUR/β -CD for 15 wks: 1 wk after the stop of DSS.	Suppression of inflammation and tumor inhibitory effect.	[88]
American Ginseng (AG)	1 i.p. AOM (10 mg/kg bw) + 3 cycles of 1% DSS in drinking water, 1 wk after AOM (a cycle consisted of 7 days of 1% DSS followed by 14 days of normal water). Strain: Male and female C57BL/6 mice.	Diet containing AG (75 ppm) for 70 days: at the same time of the start of DSS.	Suppression of colon cancer associated with colitis.	[89]
Tocopherols and Tocotrienols	2 i.p. AOM (5 mg/kg bw) at 4-day intervals + 1.5% DSS in drinking water for 1 wk. Strain: Male CF-1 mice.	Diet supplemented with 0.3% m-T (mixture of tocopherols) for 21 wks, starting 1 wk before AOM injection until the termination of the experiment.	The first comprehensive report describing simultaneous analysis of different side-chain metabolites of tocopherols and tocotrienols in mice.	[91]
Resveratrol	1 i.p. AOM (10 mg/kg bw) + 1% DSS in drinking water for 1 wk, 1 wk after AOM. Strain: Male and female C57BL/6 mice.	Diet containing Resveratrol (300 ppm) for 70 days: at the same time of the start of DSS.	Significant reduction of tumor incidence and inflammation.	[92]
2,3',4,4',5'-pentamethoxy- *trans*-stilbene (PMS)	1 i.p. AOM (10 mg/kg bw) + 2 cycles of 3% DSS in drinking water, 1 wk after AOM (a cycle consisted of 7 days of 3% DSS followed by 14 days of normal water). Strain: Balb/c mice.	Intragastric administration of PMS (25- 50 mg/kg bw) for 16 wks, starting with the AOM injection.	Suppression of colon carcinogenesis.	[93]
Zerumbone (ZER)	1 i.p. AOM (10 mg/kg bw) + 1,5%DSS in drinking water for 1 wk, 1 wk after AOM. Strain: Male Crj: CD-1 (ICR) mice.	ZER diet (100, 250, 500 ppm) for 17 wks: 1 wk after the stop of DSS.	Inhibition of adenocarcinoma occurrence and inflammation.	[94]

Table 2. (Continued)

Compound	Model and strain	Experimental protocol	Observations	References
Natural plant compounds				
Silibinin	6 i.p. AOM (5 mg/kg dose) at weekly intervals. Strain: Male A/J mice.	Silibinin (250 or 750 mg/kg/day dose, 5 days/wk) in CMC initiated 2 wks prior/after to AOM and continued for 25 wks.	Chemopreventive efficacy in colon tumorigenesis; inhibition of inflammation and angiogenesis.	[95]
Phenethyl isothiocyanate (PEITC) and dibenzoylmethane (DBM)	1 i.p. AOM (10 mg/kg bw) + 1%DSS in drinking water for 1 wk, 1 wk after AOM. Strain: Male C57BL/6 mice.	Diet supplemented with 0.05% PEITC or 1% DBM before or after AOM initiation.	Reduction of tumor incidence and multiplicity. PEITC is effective even after AOM initiation, whereas DBM is not as effective when fed after AOM initiation.	[96]
Tricin	1 i.p. AOM (10 mg/kg bw) + 1.5%DSS in drinking water for 1 wk, 1 wk after AOM. Strain: Male Crj: CD-1 mice.	Diet containing Tricin (50-250 ppm) for 70 days: at the same time of the start of DSS.	Chemopreventive efficacy in colon tumorigenesis.	[97]
MODULATION OF PHYSIOLOGICAL MOLECULES				
Selenium	1 i.p. AOM (10 mg/kg bw) once a wk for 3 wks + 2% DSS in drinking water for 1 wk, 2 wks later. Strain: Male Crj: CD-1 mice.	HFe diet (450 ppm Fe) with three different levels of Se [LSe (0.02 ppm Se), MSe (0.1 ppm Se), or HSe (0.5 ppm Se) for 24 wks.	Se supplemented diet has protective effect against colon cancer by decreasing proliferation, increasing apoptosis of tumor cells, and reducing oxidative stress in mice with high iron diet.	[100]
8-hydroxydeoxyguanosine (8-OHdG)	1 i.p. AOM (10 mg/kg bw) + 2.5%DSS in drinking water for 1 wk, 1 wk after AOM. Strain: Male Crj: C57BL/6J (IL-10 KO) mice.	Diet containing 8-OHdG (50 or 100 mg/kg/day) for 20 wks: 1 wk after the stop of DSS.	Significant inhibition if recruitment of inflammatory cells in DSS-induced colitis, and chemopreventive role in AOM/DSS-induced colitis associated cancer.	[103]
NEU3	1 i.p. AOM (10 mg/kg bw) + 1.5%DSS in drinking water for 1 wk, 1 wk after AOM. Strain: Neu3-deficient (Neu3-/-) mice.	–	The Neu3-deficient mice are less susceptible than wild-type mice to the colitis-associated colon carcinogenesis induced by AOM/DSS.	[104]

Compound	Model and strain	Experimental protocol	Observations	References
Natural plant compounds				
Compound	Model and strain	Experimental protocol	Observations	References
Interleukin-21 (IL-21)	1 i.p. AOM (10 mg/kg bw) + 4-days of 2% DSS in drinking water, 1 wk after AOM. Second i.p. injection of AOM (5 mg/kg), 1 wk after the discontinuation of DSS + 4-days of 2% DSS in drinking water, 1 wk after AOM. Strain: Male Crj: C57BL/6J mice (IL-21-/-).	–	21 blockade reduces the risk of inflammation-associated colon cancer.	[104, 105]
Peroxisome proliferator-activated receptor-γ coactivator 1-α (PGC1α)	1 i.p. AOM (12 mg/kg bw) + 2% DSS in drinking water, 5 days later, over 5 days, followed by 16 days of regular water. Cycle repeated 3 time. Strain: Male Crj: C57BL/6J mice (iPGC1α/ApcMin/+).	–	PGC1α regulates enterocyte cell fate and protects against tumorigenesis.	[106]
SYNTHETIC DRUGS				
PPAR inhibitors				
Troglitazone	1 i.p. AOM (10 mg/kg bw) + 2% DSS in drinking water for 1 wk, 1 wk after AOM. Strain: Female CD-1 (ICR) mice.	Diet containing troglitazone (0.05%) for 14 wks: 1 wk after the stop of DSS.	Suppression of the development of colonic epithelial malignancy. Induction of apoptosis.	[110]
RS5444	4 i.p. injections AOM (10 mg/kg bw) at weekly intervals. Strain: Female C57BL/6J mice.	Oral gavage of RS5444 (10 mg/kg/day) for 1 wk: prior to the initial injection of AOM.	Inhibition of early stage colon carcinogenesis.	[111]
	4 i.p. injections AOM (10 mg/kg bw) at weekly intervals. Strain: Female C57BL/6J mice.	Diet containing RS5444: 24 wks after the last AOM injection.	Decrease of about 30% in tumor incidence.	[112]
SK1 inhibitors				
ABC294640	1 i.p. AOM (10 mg/kg bw) + 1% DSS in drinking water for 1 wk, 1 wk after AOM. Strain: Female C57BL/6J mice.	Daily i.p. injection of ABC294640 (20-50 mg/kg bw) 5 days per week until the end of the experiment on Day 70.	Dose-dependent decrease in tumor incidence and multiplicity. Suppression of colitis.	[113]
COX-2 inhibitors				

Table 2. (Continued)

Compound	Model and strain	Experimental protocol	Observations	References
Natural plant compounds				
Sulfasalazine	1 i.p. AOM (8 mg/kg bw) + 3 cycles of 3% DSS in drinking water, 1 wk after AOM (a cycle consisted of 7 days of 3% DSS followed by 7 days of distilled water). Strain: Female CBA/J mice.	Diet containing Sulfasalazine (500 mg in 1 kg of diet) for 15 wks.	Reduction of tumorous regions with high-grade dysplasia.	[114]
5-ASA	1 i.p. AOM (7.4 mg/kg bw) + 3 cycles of 4% DSS in drinking water, 2 wks after AOM (a cycle consisted of 7 days of 4% DSS followed by 14 days of normal water). Strain: Female Swiss Webster mice.	ASA (75, 150 or 225 mg/kg bw) in drinking water: 1 wk after the AOM injection, for 18 wks.	Reduction of susceptibility for colitis associated CRC neoplasia.	[115]
Sulfasalazine	1 i.p. AOM (10 mg/kg bw) + 1% DSS in drinking water for 1 wk, 1 wk after AOM. Strain: Male Crj:CD-1 (ICR) mice.	Diet containing Sulfasalazine (0.05%) for 15 wks: 1 wk after the stop of DSS.	Weak suppressive effect on tumor formation.	[116]
UDCA	1 i.p. AOM (10 mg/kg bw) + 1% DSS in drinking water for 1 wk, 1 wk after AOM Strain: Male Crj:CD-1 (ICR) mice.	Diet containing UDCA (0.016%, 0.08%, 0.4%) for 17 wks: 1 wk after the stop of DSS.	Significantly inhibition of the multiplicity of colonic adenocarcinoma.	[116]
5-ASA derivate 2-14	1 i.p. AOM (7.4 mg/kg bw) + 3 cycles of 4% DSS in drinking water, 2 wks after AOM (a cycle consisted of 7 days of 4% DSS followed by 14 days of normal water). Strain: Balb/c mice.	Daily i.p. injection of 2-14 (8 mg/kg mouse/day): 2 wks after the last DSS administration.	Significant reduction of flat and polypoid neoplastic lesions. No effects on normal colon epithelial cells.	[117]
Nimesulide	1 i.p. AOM (10 mg/kg bw) + 2% DSS in drinking water for 1 wk, 1 wk after AOM. Strain: Female CD-1 (ICR) mice.	Diet containing Nimesulide (0.04%) for 14 wks: 1 wk after the stop of DSS.	Suppression of the development of colonic epithelial malignancy Inhibition of colitis.	[118]
HDAC inhibitors				
SAHA (suberyolanilide hydroxamic acid) and ITF2357	1 i.p. AOM (12.5 mg/kg bw) + 3 cycles of 3.5% DSS in drinking water, 5 days after AOM (a cycle consisted of 5 days of 3.5% DSS followed by 14 days of distilled water). Strain: C57BL/6J mice.	Oral gavage of SAHA (50 mg/kg) and ITF2357 (10 mg/kg) once daily during the entire experimental time course (50 days): given simultaneously with the start of DSS.	Prevention of inflammation-induced tumourigenesis.	[119]

AOM: azoxymethane; DSS: dextran sodium sulphate; i.p. injection: intraperitoneal injection; 5-ASA: 5-aminosalicylic acid; UDCA: ursodeoxycholic acid; PPARs: peroxisome proliferator-activated receptors; CMC: carboxymethyl cellulose; wk: week.

Kohno *et al.* [121] reported that the suppressive effects of sulfasalazine on CRC were relatively weak when the drug was given in the promotion/progression phase of disease development. This discrepancy may be due to differences in experimental protocols and the murine strains used. Kohno *et al.* also reported that treatment with ursodeoxycholic acid (UDCA) resulted in inhibition of AOM/DSS-induced CRC in mice, without causing any adverse effects.

Finally, a novel 5-ASA derivative called '5-ASA derivative 2-14' seems to be 10-fold more potent than 5-ASA in inhibiting CRC cell proliferation [122].

Besides 5-ASA and its derivatives, selective COX-2 inhibitors have been tested in the colorectal carcinogenesis animal model. Particularly, nimesulide (4-nitro-2-phenoxy-methanesulfonanilide), a selective inhibitor of COX-2, effectively inhibited AOM/DSS-induced colonic carcinogenesis in mice [123]. The suppressive effects of nimesulide on the development of colonic adenocarcinoma correlates well with the inhibition of cell proliferation activity, induction of apoptosis, and the lower immunoreactivity of β-catenin, COX-2, iNOS, and nitrotyrosine in colonic malignancies. These data suggest that nimesulide could be applied as an effective chemopreventor of both sporadic and IBD-associated colorectal carcinogenesis.

HDAC inhibitors - Given the generally known antiproliferative capacity of histone deacetylase (HDAC) inhibitors on intestinal inflammation, a strong tumor preventing capacity of HDAC inhibition has been assumed in cases where chronic inflammation is clearly associated with a subsequent tumorigenesis.

Experimental colitis in mice represents an excellent *in vivo* model to define the specific cell populations and target tissues modulated by inhibitors of HDAC.

At this purpose, HDAC inhibitors have been successfully tested in the AOM/DSS model, where oral administration of either suberyolanilide hydroxamic acid (SAHA) or ITF2357 results in an amelioration in this model, as indicated by a significantly attenuation of both colitis and tumor growth and development [124].

Conclusion

People living in Western countries have a 35-50% chance of getting some type of cancer in their lifetime. Environmental factors and lifestyle are now known to be largely responsible for this problem. In order to plan strategies and efforts addressed to prevent the disease, we first need to understand it by investigating its mechanisms of development.

Because human studies are extremely long and costly, stringent preliminary studies in animal models, mimicking the development of the disease in humans, are strongly required.

Experimental rodent models are essential tools for investigating development and pathogenesis of CRC. In fact, the molecular characterization of genetic and epigenetic alterations during the steps of a spontaneously induced colon cancer, can open new perspectives for diagnostic, prognostic and predictive studies and also for preclinical protocols of novel therapeutic options to translate in the clinical practice.

Among the variety of available CRC animal models, the choice of a model which reproduces the steps occurring in humans is a crucial point. Inflammation-dependent CRC tumor growth in mouse models can be investigated by AOM/DSS treated mice, combining the administration of Azoxymethane with the inflammatory agent Dextran Sodium Sulfate in drinking water, which causes rapid growth of multiple colon tumors per mouse within 10 weeks. As explained in this chapter such model offers lots of advantages compared to other kinds of chemically-induced models, as high potency and reproducibility, simple mode of application, short time and low costs. In contrast to other models of CRC, tumors induced by AOM and promoted through a local inflammation provoked by DSS are very frequent in the distal part of the colon, which resembles the predominant localization of spontaneous CRC with high hystopathological and molecular correspondence with human colon carcinogenesis mediated by inflammation conditions. For this reason, the choice of this experimental platform is particularly applicable when the focus of the study are the tumor progression mechanisms driven by colitis.

Moreover, chemoprevention studies as well as investigation of novel diagnostic, prognostic and predictive markers to use in clinical practice can be also successfully performed in this valuable model as tumor development is predictable and consistent, with a high incidence of affected animals in a narrow time frame.

In the future, novel and more sophisticated molecular tools and genetic strategies coupled with further improvements of the AOM/DSS model, might enable to define new aspects of CRCs, such as the molecular networks altered in the earliest phase of this neoplastic disease or the identification of the genetic and epigenetic events, still partially unknown, that act in the pre-neoplastic phase of colon which are fundamental in CRC development.

Acknowledgment

This work has been kindly revised by Prof SA Ciafré, Dept. of Biomedicine and Prevention, School of Medicine, University of Rome Tor Vergata.

References

[1] Haggar, FA; Boushey, RP. Colorectal Cancer Epidemiology: Incidence, Mortality, Survival, and Risk Factors. *Clin. Colon Rectal Surg.* 2009,22,191–197.

[2] van Hogezand, RA; Eichhorn, RF; Choudry, A; Veenendaal, RA; Lamers, BHW. Malignancies in inflammatory bowel disease: fact or fiction? *Scand. J. Gastroenterol. Suppl.* 2002,235,48–53.

[3] Gala, M; Chung, DC. Hereditary colon cancer syndromes. *Semin. Oncol.* 2011;38,490–9.

[4] Al-Sohaily, S; Biankin, A; Leong, R; Kohonen-Corish, M; Warusavitarne, J. Molecular pathways in colorectal cancer. *J. Gastroenterol. Hepatol.* 2012,27,1423–1431.

[5] Friedman, E; Urmacher, C; Winawer, S. A model for human colon carcinoma evolution based on the differential response of cultured preneoplastic, premalignant, and malignant cells to 12-O-tetradecanoylphorbol-13-acetate. *Cancer Res.* 1984,44,1568–78.

[6] Fodde, R; Smits, R. Disease model: familial adenomatous polyposis. *Trends Mol. Med.* 2001,7,369–73.

[7] Takaku, K; Sonoshita, M; Sasaki, N; Uozumi, N; Doi, Y; Shimizu, T; Taketo, MM. Suppression of intestinal polyposis in Apc (delta 716) knockout mice by an additional mutation in the cytosolic phospholipase A(2) gene. *J. Biol. Chem.* 2000,275,34013–6.

[8] Oshima, M; Dinchuk, JE; Kargman, SL; Oshima, H; Hancock, B; Kwong, E; Trzaskos, JM; Evans, JF; Taketo, MM. Suppression of intestinal polyposis in Apc delta716 knockout mice by inhibition of cyclooxygenase 2 (COX-2). *Cell* 1996,87,803–9.

[9] Seno, H; Oshima, M; Ishikawa, TO; Oshima, H; Takaku, K; Chiba, T; Narumiya, S; Taketo, MM. Cyclooxygenase 2- and prostaglandin E(2) receptor EP(2)-dependent angiogenesis in Apc(Delta716) mouse intestinal polyps. *Cancer Res.* 2002,62,506–11.

[10] Heyer, J; Yang, K; Lipkin, M; Edelmann, W; Kucherlapati R. Mouse models for colorectal cancer. *Oncogene* 1999,18,5325–33.

[11] Garofalo, A; Chirivi, RG; Scanziani, E; Mayo, JG; Vecchi, A; Giavazzi, R. Comparative study on the metastatic behavior of human tumors in nude, beige/nude/xid and severe combined immunodeficient mice. *Invasion Metastasis* 1993,13,82–91.

[12] Zigmond, E; Halpern, Z; Elinav, E; Brazowski, E; Jung, S; Varol, C. Utilization of Murine Colonoscopy for Orthotopic Implantation of Colorectal Cancer. *PLoS ONE* 2011,6,e28858.

[13] Ito, N; Hasegawa, R; Sano, M; Tamano, S; Esumi, H; Takayama, S; Sugimura, T. A new colon and mammary carcinogen in cooked food, 2-amino-1-methyl-6-phenylimidazo [4,5-b]pyridine (PhIP). *Carcinogenesis* 1991, 12, 1503–150.

[14] Kato, T; Ohgaki, H; Hasegawa, H; Sato, S; Takayama, S; Sugimura T. Carcinogenicity in rats of a mutagenic compound, 2-amino-3,8-dimethylimidazo [4,5-f]quinoxaline. *Carcinogenesis* 1988, 9,71–73.

[15] Hasegawa, R; Sano, M; Tamano, S; Imaida, K; Shirai, T; Nagao, M; Sugimura, T; Ito, N. Dose-dependence of 2-amino-1-methyl-6-phenylimidazo [4,5-b]-pyridine (PhIP) carcinogenicity in rats. *Carcinogenesis* 1993,14,2553–7.

[16] Reddy, BS; Rivenson, A. Inhibitory effect of Bifidobacterium longum on colon, mammary, and liver carcinogenesis induced by 2-amino-3-methylimidazo [4,5-f] quinoline, a food mutagen. *Cancer Res.* 1993,53,3914–8.

[17] Doi, K; Wanibuchi, H; Salim, EI; Morimura, K; Kinoshita, A; Kudoh, S; Hirata, K; Yoshikawa, J; Fukushima, S. Lack of large intestinal carcinogenicity of 2-amino-1-methyl-6-phenylimidazo [4,5-b] pyridine at low doses in rats initiated with azoxymethane. *Int. J. Cancer* 2005,115,870–8.

[18] Kobaek-Larsen, M; Thorup, I; Diederichsen, A; Fenger, C; Hoitinga, MR. Review of colorectal cancer and its metastases in rodent models: comparative aspects with those in humans. *Comp. Med.* 2000,50,16–26.

[19] Walpole, A; Williams, MH; Roberts, DC. The carcinogenic action of 4-aminodiphenyl and 3:2'-dimethyl-4-amino-diphenyl. *Br. J. Ind. Med.* 1952,9,255–63.

[20] Reddy, BS; Ohmori, T. Effect of intestinal microflora and dietary fat on 3,2'-dimethyl-4-aminobiphenyl-induced colon carcinogenesis in F344 rats. *Cancer Res.* 1981,41,1363–7.

[21] Narisawa, T; Magadia, NE; Weisburger, JH; Wynder, EL. Promoting effect of bile acids on colon carcinogenesis after intrarectal instillation of N-methyl-N'-nitro-N-nitrosoguanidine in rats. *J. Natl. Cancer Inst.* 1974,53,1093–7.

[22] Heijstek MW, Kranenburg O, Borel Rinkes IH. Mouse models of colorectal cancer and liver metastases. *Dig. Surg.* 2005,22,16–25.

[23] Laqueur, GL, Mickelsen, O; Whiting, MG; Kurland, LT. Carcinogenic Properties of Nuts from Cycas Circinalis L. Indigenous to Guam. *J. Natl. Cancer Inst.* 1963,31,919–51.

[24] Martin, MS; Martin, F, Michiels, R; Bastien, H; Justrabo, E; Bordes, M; Viry, B. An experimental model for cancer of the colon and rectum. Intestinal carcinoma induced in the rat 1,2-dimethylhydrazine. *Digestion* 1973,8,22–34.

[25] Ward, JM. Morphogenesis of chemically induced neoplasms of the colon and small intestine in rats. *Lab. Invest* 1974,30,505–13.

[26] Sohn, OS; Fiala, ES; Requeijo, SP; Weisburger, JH; Gonzalez, FJ. Differential effects of CYP2E1 status on the metabolic activation of the colon carcinogens azoxymethane and methylazoxymethanol *Cancer Res.* 2001,61,8435–40.

[27] Papanikolaou, A; Wang, QS; Delker, DA; Rosenberg, DW. Azoxymethane-induced colon tumors and aberrant crypt foci in mice of different genetic susceptibility. *Cancer Lett.* 1998,130,29–34.

[28] Papanikolaou, A; Wang, QS; Mulherkar, R; Bolt, A; Rosenberg, DW. Expression analysis of the group IIA secretory phospholipase A(2) in mice with differential susceptibility to azoxymethane-induced colon tumorigenesis. *Carcinogenesis* 2000,21,133–8.

[29] Tanaka, T; Kohno, H; Suzuki, R; Yamada, Y; Sugie, S; Mori, H. A novel inflammation related mouse colon carcinogenesis model induced by azoxymethane and dextran sodium sulfate. *Cancer Sci.* 2003,94,965–73.

[30] De Robertis, M; Massi, E; Poeta, ML; Carotti, S; Morini, S; Cecchetelli, L; Signori, E; Fazio, VM. The AOM/DSS murine model for the study of colon carcinogenesis: From pathways to diagnosis and therapy studies. *J. Carcinog.* 2011,24,10–9.

[31] Neufert, C; Becker, C; Neurath, MF. An inducible mouse model of colon carcinogenesis for the analysis of sporadic and inflammation-driven tumor progression. *Nat. Protoc.* 2007,2,1998–2004.

[32] Clapp, NK; Henke, MA; London, JF; Shock TL. Enhancement of 1,2-dimethylhydrazine-induced large bowel tumorigenesis in Balb/c mice by corn, soybean, and wheat brans. *Nutr. Cancer* 1984,6,77–85.

[33] Hata, K; Yamada, Y; Kuno, T; Hirose, Y; Hara, A; Qiang, SH; Mori, H. Tumor formation is correlated with expression of beta-catenin-accumulated crypts in azoxymethane-induced colon carcinogenesis in mice. *Cancer Sci.* 2004,95,316–20.

[34] Papanikolaou, A; Wang, QS; Papanikolaou, D; Whiteley, HE; Rosenberg, DW. Sequential and morphological analyses of aberrant crypt foci formation in mice of differing susceptibility to azoxymethane-induced colon carcinogenesis. *Carcinogenesis* 2000,21,1567–72.

[35] Bissahoyo, A; Pearsall, RS; Hanlon, K; Amann, V; Hicks, D; Godfrey, VL; Threadqill, DW. Azoxymethane is a genetic background-dependent colorectal tumor initiator and promoter in mice: effects of dose, route, and diet. *Toxicol. Sci.* 2005,88,340–5.

[36] Okayasu, I; Ohkusa, T; Kajiura, K; Kanno, J; Sakamoto S. Promotion of colorectal neoplasia in experimental murine ulcerative colitis. *Gut* 1996,39,87–92.

[37] Becker, C; Fantini, MC; Schramm, C; Lehr, HA; Wirtz, S; Nikolaev, A; Burg, J; Strand, S; Kiesslich, R; Huber, S; Ito, H; Nishimoto, N; Yoshizaki, K; Kishimoto, T; Galle, PR; Blessing, M; Rose-John S, Neurath MF. TGF-beta suppresses tumor

progression in colon cancer by inhibition of IL-6 trans-signaling. *Immunity* 2004,21,491–501.

[38] Becker, C; Fantini, MC; Wirtz, S; Nikolaev, A; Kiesslich, R; Lehr, HA; Galle, PR; Neurath, MF. In vivoimagingofcolitisandcolon cancerdevelopmentinmice using high resolution chromoendoscopy. *Gut* 2005,54,950–4.

[39] Rosenberg, DW; Giardina, C; Tanaka, T. Mouse models for the study of colon carcinogenesis. *Carcinogenesis* 2009,30,183–96.

[40] Salim, EI; Wanibuchi, H; Morimura, K; Murai, T; Makino, S; Nomura, T; Fukushima, S. Induction of tumors in the colon and liver of the immunodeficient (SCID) mouse by 2-amino-3-methylimidazo [4,5-f]quinoline (IQ)-modulation by long-chain fatty acids. *Carcinogenesis* 2002,23,1519–29.

[41] Mølck, AM; Meyer, O; Kristiansen, E; Thorup, I. IQ (2-amino-3-methylimidazo [4,5-f]quinoline)-induced aberrant crypt foci and colorectal tumour development in rats fed two different carbohydrate diets. *Eur. J. Cancer Prev.* 2001,10,501–6.

[42] Ito, N; Hasegawa, R; Imaida, K; Tamano, S; Hagiwara, A; Hirose, M; Shirai, T. Carcinogenicity of 2-amino-1-methyl-6-phenylimidazo [4,5-b]pyridine (PhIP) in the rat. *Mutat Res.* 1997,376,107–14.

[43] Wang, R; Dashwood, WM; Löhr, CV; Fischer, KA; Pereira, CB; Louderback, M; Nakagama, H; Bailey, GS; Williams, DE; Dashwood, RH. Protective versus promotional effects of white tea and caffeine on PhIP-induced tumorigenesis and β-catenin expression in the rat. *Carcinogenesis* 2008,29,834–839.

[44] Nakagama, H; Ochiai, M; Ubagai, T; Tajima, R; Fujiwara, K; Sugimura, T; Nagao, M. A rat colon cancer model induced by 2-amino-1-methyl-6-phenylimidazo [4,5-b]pyridine, PhIP. *Mutat Res.* 2002,506-507,137–44.

[45] Yang, J; Shikata, N; Mizuoka, H; Tsubura, A. Colon carcinogenesis in shrews by intrarectal infusion of N-methyl-N-nitrosourea. *Cance Lett.* 1996,110,105–112.

[46] Zusman, I; Zimber, A; Nyska, A. Role of morphological methods in the analysis of chemically induced colon cancer in rats. *Acta Anat. Basel* 1991,142,351–356.

[47] Nambiar, PR; Girnun, G; Lillo, NA; Guda, K; Whiteley, HE; Rosenberg, DW. Preliminary analysis of azoxymethane induced colon tumors in inbred mice commonly used as transgenic/knockout progenitors. *Int. J. Oncol.* 2003,22,145–50.

[48] Kim, YJ; Hong, KS; Chung, JW; Kim, JH; Hahm, KB. Prevention of colitis-associated carcinogenesis with infliximab. *Cancer Prevention Research* 2010,3,1314–1333.

[49] Nishikawa, A; Imazawa, T; Kuroiwa, Y; Kitamura, Y; Kanki, K; Ishii; Y; Umemura, T; Hirose, M. Induction of colon tumors in C57BL/6J mice fed MeIQx, IQ, or PhIP followed by dextran sulfate sodium. *Toxicol. Sci. Toxicol. Sci.* 2005,84,243–8.

[50] Meira, LB; Bugni, JM; Green, SL; Lee, CW; Pang, B; Borenshtein, D; Rickman, BH; Rogers, AB; Moroski-Erkul, CA; McFaline, JL; Schauer, DB; Dedon, PC; Fox, JG; Samson, LD. DNA damage induced by chronic inflammation contributes to colon carcinogenesis in mice. *J. Clin. Invest.* 2008,118,2516–25.

[51] Suzuki, R; Kohno, H; Sugie, S; Nakagama, H; Tanaka, T. Strain differences in the susceptibility to azoxymethane and dextran sodium sulfate-induced colon carcinogenesis in mice. *Carcinogenesis* 2006,27,162–9.

[52] Bird, RP; Good, CK. The significance of aberrant crypt foci in understanding the pathogenesis of colon cancer. *Toxicol. Lett.* 2000, 112,395–402.

[53] Yamada, Y; Yoshimi, N; Hirose, Y; Matsunaga, K; Katayama, M; Sakata, K; Shimizu, M; Kuno, T; Mori, H. Sequential analysis of morphological and biological properties of beta-catenin-accumulated crypts, provable premalignant lesions independent of aberrant crypt foci in rat colon carcinogenesis. *Cancer Res.* 2001,61,1874–8.

[54] Caderni, G; Femia, AP; Giannini, A; Favuzza, A; Luceri, C; Salvadori, M; Dolara, P. Identification of mucin-depleted foci in the unsectioned colon of azoxymethane-treated rats: correlation with carcinogenesis. *Cancer Res.* 2003,63,2388–92.

[55] Paulsen, JE; Løberg, EM; Olstørn, HB; Knutsen, H; Steffensen, IL; Alexander, J. Flat dysplastic aberrant crypt foci are related to tumorigenesis in the colon of azoxymethane-treated rat. *Cancer Res.* 2005,65,121–9.

[56] Yasui, Y; Tanaka T. Protein expression analysis of inflammation-related colon carcinogenesis. *J. Carcinog.* 2009,8,10.

[57] Gerling, M; Glauben, R; Habermann, JK; Kuhl, AA; Loddenkemper, C; Lehr, AH; Zeitz, M; Siegmund, B. Characterization of Chromosomal Instability in Murine Colitis-Associated Colorectal Cancer. *PLoS ONE* 2011,6,e22114.

[58] Cooper, HS; Murthy, S; Kido, K; Yoshitake, H; Flanigan, A. Dysplasia and cancer in the dextran sulfate sodium mouse colitis model. Relevance to colitisassociated neoplasia in the human: a study of histopathology, B-catenin and p53 expression and the role of inflammation. *Carcinogenesis* 2000,21,757–68.

[59] Kohno, H; Suzuki, R; Sugie, S; Tanaka, T. Beta-Catenin mutations in a mouse model of inflammation-related colon carcinogenesis induced by 1,2-dimethylhydrazine and dextran sodium sulfate. *Cancer Sci.* 2005,96,69–76.

[60] Svec, J; Ergang, P; Mandys, V; Kment, M; Pácha, J. Expression profiles of proliferative and antiapoptotic genes in sporadic and colitis-related mouse colon cancer models. *Int. J. Exp. Path* 2010,91,44–53.

[61] Jacoby, RF; Llor, X; Teng, BB; Davidson, NO; Brasitus, TA. Mutations in the K-ras oncogene induced by 1,2-dimethylhydrazine in preneoplastic and neoplastic rat colonic mucosa. *J. Clin. Invest.* 1991,87,624–30.

[62] Yekkala, K; Baudino, TA. Inhibition of intestinal polyposis with reduced angiogenesis in ApcMin/+ mice due to decreases in c-Myc expression. *Mol. Cancer Res.* 2007,5,1296–303.

[63] Suzuki, R; Miyamoto, S; Yasui, Y; Sugie, S; Tanaka, T. Global gene expression analysis of the mouse colonic mucosa treated with azoxymethane and dextran sodium sulfate. *BMC Cancer* 2007,7,84.

[64] Choi, J; Southworth, LK; Sarin, KY; Venteicher, AS; Ma, W; Chang, W; Cheung, P; Jun, S; Artandi, MK; Shah, N; Kim, SK; Artandi, SE. TERT promotes epithelial proliferation through transcriptional control of a Myc- and Wnt-related developmental program. *PLoS Genet* 2008,4,e10.

[65] Becker, C; Fantini, MC; Neurath, MF. TGF-beta as a T cell regulator in colitis and colon cancer. *Cytokine Growth Factor Rev.* 2006,17,97–106.

[66] DuBois, RN; Radhika, A; Reddy, BS; Entingh, AJ. Increased cyclooxygenase-2 levels in carcinogen-induced rat colonic tumors. *Gastroenterology* 1996,110,1259–1262.

[67] Guda, K; Giardina, C; Nambiar, P; Cui, H; Rosenberg, DW. Aberrant transforming growth factor-β signaling in azoxymethane-induced mouse colon tumors. *Molecular Carcinogenesis* 2001,31, 204–213.

[68] Relan, NK; Saeed, A; Ponduri, K; Fligiel, SEG; Dutta, S; Majumdar, APN. Identification and evaluation of the role of endogenous tyrosine kinases in azoxymethane induction of proliferative processes in the colonic mucosa of rats. *Biochimica et Biophysica Acta* 1995, 1244,2-3,368–376.

[69] Sinicrope, FA; Gill, S. Role of cyclooxygenase-2 in colorectal cancer. *Cancer Metastasis Rev.* 2004,23,63–75.

[70] Kim, HS; Kundu, JK; Le, JS; Oh, TY; Na, HK; Surh, YJ. Chemopreventive effects of the standardized extract (DA-9601) of Artemisia asiatica on azoxymethaneinitiated and dextran sulfate sodium-promoted mouse colon carcinogenesis. *Nutr. Cancer* 2008,60,90–7.

[71] Seril, DN; Liao, J; Yang, GY. Colorectal carcinoma development in inducible nitric oxide synthase-deficient mice with dextran sulfate sodium-induced ulcerative colitis. *Mol. Carcinog.* 2007,46,341–53.

[72] Kohno, H; Suzuki, R; Curini, M; Epifano, F; Maltese, F; Gonzales, SP; Tanaka, T. Dietary administration with prenyloxycoumarins, auraptene and collinin, inhibits colitis-related colon carcinogenesis in mice. *Int. J. Cancer* 2006,118,2936–42.

[73] Takahashi, M; Mutoh, M; Kawamori, T; Sugimura, T; Wakabayashi, K. Altered expression of beta-catenin, inducible nitric oxide synthase and cyclooxygenase-2 in azoxymethane-induced rat colon carcinogenesis. *Carcinogenesis* 2000,21,1319–27.

[74] Nambiar, PR; Giardina, C; Guda, K; Aizu, W; Raja, R; Rosenberg, DW. Role of the alternating reading frame (P19)-p53 pathway in an in vivo murine colon tumor model. *Cancer Res.* 2002,62,3667–74.

[75] Gaudet, F; Hodgson, JG; Eden, A; Jackson-Grusby, L; Dausman, J; Gra, JW; Leonhardt, H; Jaenisch, R. Induction of tumors in mice by genomic hypomethylation. *Science* 2003,300,489–92.

[76] Borinstein, SC; Conerly, M; Dzieciatkowski, S; Biswas, S; Washington, MK; Trobridge, P; Henikoff, S; Grady, WM. Aberrant DNA methylation occurs in colon neoplasms arising in the azoxymethane colon cancer model. *Mol. Carcinog.* 2010,49,94–103.

[77] Nagamine, CM; Rogers, AB; Fox, JG; Schauer, DB. Helicobacter hepaticus promotes azoxymethane-initiated colon tumorigenesis in BALB/c-IL10-deficient mice. *International Journal of Cancer* 2008,122,832–838.

[78] Okayasu, I; Yamada, M; Mikami, T; Yoshida, T; Kanno, J; Ohkusa, T. Dysplasia and carcinoma development in a repeated dextran sulfate sodium-induced colitis model. *J. Gastroenterol. Hepatol.* 2002,17,1078–83.

[79] Greten, FR; Karin, M. The IKK/NF-kappaB activation pathway-a target for prevention and treatment of cancer. *Cancer Lett.* 2004,206,193–9.

[80] Paradisi, A; Maisse, C; Bernet, A; Coissieux, MM; Maccarrone, M; Scoazec, JY; Mehlen, P.NF-kappaB regulates netrin-1 expression and affects the conditional tumor suppressive activity of the netrin-1 receptors. *Gastroenterology*2008,135,1248–57.

[81] Popivanova, BK; Kitamura, K; Wu, Y; Kondo, T; Kagaya, T; Kaneko, S; Oshima, M; Fujii, C; Mukaida, N. Blocking TNF-alpha in mice reduces colorectal carcinogenesis associated with chronic colitis. *J. Clin. Invest.* 2008,118,560–70.

[82] Balkwill, F. Tumour necrosis factor and cancer. *Nat. Rev. Cancer* 2009,9,361–71.

[83] Becker, C; Fantini, MC; Schramm, C; Lehr, HA; Wirtz, S; Nikolaev, A; Burg, J;

[84] Strand, S; Kiesslich, R; Huber, S; Ito, H; Nishimoto, N; Yoshizaki, K; Kishimoto, T; Galle, PR; Blessing, M; Rose-John, S; Neurath, MF. TGF-βsuppresses tumor progression in colon cancer by inhibition of IL-6 trans-signaling," *Immunity* 2004, 21, 491–501.

[85] Stolfi, C; Rizzo, A; Franzè, E; Rotondi, A; Fantini, MC; Sarra, M; Caruso, R; Monteleone, I; Sileri, P; Franceschilli, L; Caprioli, F; Ferrero, S; MacDonald, TT; Pallone, F; Monteleone G. Involvement of interleukin-21 in the regulation of colitis-associated colon cancer. *J. Exp. Med.* 2011,208,2279–2290.

[86] Hanada, T; Kobayashi, T; Chinen, T; Saeki, K; Takaki, H; Koga, K; Minoda, Y; Sanada, T; Yoshioka, T; Mimata, H; Kato, S; Yoshimura, A. IFNgamma-dependent, spontaneous development of colorectal carcinomas in SOCS1-deficient mice. *J. Exp. Med.* 2006,203,1391–7.

[87] Vetrano, S; Borroni, EM; Sarukhan, A; Savino, B; Bonecchi, R; Correale, C; Arena, V; Fantini, M; Roncalli, M; Malesci, A; Mantovani, A; Locati, M; Danese, S. The lymphatic system controls intestinal inflammation and inflammation-associated Colon Cancer through the chemokine decoy receptor D6. *Gut* 2010,59,197–206.

[88] Fukata, M; Chen, A; Vamadevan, AS; Cohen, J; Breglio, K; Krishnareddy, S; Hsu, D; Xu, R; Harpaz, N; Dannenberg, AJ; Subbaramaiah, K; Cooper, HS; Itzkowitz, SH; Abreu, MT. Toll-like receptor-4 promotes the development of colitis-associated colorectal tumors. *Gastroenterology*. 2007,133,1869–1881.

[89] Fukata, M; Chen, A; Klepper, A; Krishnareddy, S; Vamadevan, AS; Thomas, LS; Xu, R; Inoue, H; Arditi, M; Dannenberg, AJ; Abreu, MT. Cox-2 is regulated by Toll-like receptor-4 (TLR4) signaling: role in proliferation and apoptosis in the intestine. *Gastroenterology* 2006,131,862–877.

[90] Hernandez, Y; Sotolongo, J; Breglio, K; Conduah, D; Chen, A; Xu, R; Hsu, D; Ungaro, R; Hayes, LA; Pastorini, C; Abreu, MT; Fukata, M. The role of prostaglandin E2(PGE 2) in Toll-like receptor 4 (TLR4)-mediated colitis-associated neoplasia. *BMC Gastroenterology* 2010,10,82.

[91] Salcedo, R; Worschech, A; Cardone, M; Jones, Y; Gyulai, Z; Dai, RM; Wang, E; Ma, W; Haines, D; O'hUigin, C; Marincola, FM; Trinchieri G. MyD88-mediated signaling prevents development of adenocarcinomas of the colon: role of interleukin 18. *J. Exp. Med.* Vol 2010,207,1625–1636.

[92] Garlanda, C; Riva, F; Veliz, T; Polentarutti, N; Pasqualini, F; Radaelli, E; Sironi, M; Nebuloni, M; Zorini, EO; Scanziani, E; Mantovani, A. Increased susceptibility to colitisassociated cancer of mice lacking TIR8, an inhibitory member of the interleukin-1 receptor family. *Cancer Res.* 2007,67,6017–6021.

[93] Liao, J; Seril, DN; Lu, GG; Zhang, M; Toyokuni, S; Yang, AL; Yang, GY. Increased susceptibility of chronic ulcerative colitis-induced carcinoma development in DNA repair enzyme Ogg1 deficient mice. *Mol. Carcinog.* 2008,47,638–646.

[94] Tanaka, T; de Azevedo, MB; Durán, N; Alderete, JB; Epifano, F; Genovese, S; Tanaka, M; Tanaka, T; Curini, M. Colorectal cancer chemoprevention by 2 beta-cyclodextrin inclusion compounds of auraptene and 4'-geranyloxyferulic acid. *Int. J. Cancer* 2010,126,830–40.

[95] Cui, X; Jin, Y; Poudyal, D; Chumanevich, AA; Davis, T; Windust, A; Hofseth, A; Wu, W; Habiger, J; Pena, E; Wood, P; Nagarkatti, M; Nagarkatti, PS; Hofseth, L. Mechanistic insight into the ability of American ginseng to suppress colon cancer associated with colitis. *Carcinogenesis* 2010,31,1734–41.

[96] Dougherty, U; Mustafi, R; Wang, Y; Musch, MW; Wang, CZ; Konda, VJ; Kulkarni, A; Hart, J; Dawson, G; Kim, KE; Yuan, CS; Chang, EB; Bissonnette, M. American ginseng suppresses Western diet-promoted tumorigenesis in model of inflammation-associated colon cancer: role of EGFR. *BMC Complement Altern Med.* 2011,11,11.

[97] Zhao, Y; Lee, MJ; Cheung, C; Ju, JH; Chen, YK; Liu, B; Hu, LQ; Yang, CS. Analysis of Multiple Metabolites of Tocopherols andTocotrienols in Mice and Humans. *J. Agric. Food Chem.* 2010,58,4844–4852.

[98] Cui, X; Jin, Y; Hofseth, AB; Pena, E; Habiger, J; Chumanevich, A; Poudyal, D; Nagarkatti, M; Nagarkatti, PS; Singh, UP; Hofseth, LJ. Resveratrol suppresses colitis and colon cancer associated with colitis. *Cancer Prev. Res.* (Phila) 2010,3,549–559.

[99] Li, H; Wu, WK; Li, ZJ; Chan, KM; Wong, CC; Ye, CG; Yu, L; Sung, JJ; Cho, CH; Wang, M. 2,3',4,4',5'-Pentamethoxy-trans-stilbene, a resveratrol derivative, inhibits colitis-associated colorectal carcinogenesis in mice. *Br. J. Pharmacol.* 2010,160,1352–61.

[100] Murakami, A; Takahashi, D; Kinoshita, T; Koshimizu, K; Kim, HW; Yoshihiro, A; Nakamura, Y; Jiwajinda, S; Terao, J; Ohigashi, H. Zerumbone, a Southeast Asian ginger sesquiterpene, markedly suppresses free radical generation, proinflammatory protein production, and cancer cell proliferation accompanied by apoptosis: the alpha, beta-unsaturated carbonyl group is a prerequisite. *Carcinogenesis.* 2002,23,795–802.

[101] Ravichandran, K; Velmurugan, B; Gu, M; Singh, RP; Agarwal, R. Inhibitory effect of silibinin against azoxymethane-induced colon tumorigenesis in A/J Mice. *Clin. Cancer Res.* 2010,16,4595–606.

[102] Cheung, KL; Khor, TO; Huang, MT; Kong, AN. Differential in vivo mechanism of chemoprevention of tumor formation in azoxymethane/dextran sodium sulfate mice by PEITC and DBM. *Carcinogenesis* 2010,31,880–5.

[103] Oyama, T; Yasui, Y; Sugie, S; Koketsu, M; Watanabe, K; Tanaka, T. Dietary tricin suppresses inflammation-related colon carcinogenesis in male Crj: CD-1 mice. *Cancer Prev. Res.* (Phila) 2009,2,1031–8.

[104] Feng, Y; Finley, JW; Davis, CD; Becker, WK; Fretland, AJ; Hein, DW. Dietary selenium reduces the formation of aberrant crypts in rats administered 3,2'-dimethyl-4-aminobiphenyl. *Toxicol. Appl. Pharmacol.* 1999,157,36–42.

[105] Finley, JW; Davis, CD. Selenium (Se) from high-selenium broccoli is utilized differently than selenite, selenate and selenomethionine, but is more effective in inhibiting colon carcinogenesis. *Biofactors* 2001, 14,191–196.

[106] Kim, JH; Hue, JJ; Kang, BS; Park, H; Nam, SY; Yun, YW; Kim, JS; Lee, BJ. Effects of selenium on colon carcinogenesis induced by azoxymethane and dextran sodium sulfate in mouse model with high-iron diet. *Lab. Anim. Res.* 2011,27,9–18.

[107] Krehl, S; Loewinger, M; Florian, S; Kipp, AP; Banning, A; Wessjohann, LA; Brauer, MN; Iori, R; Esworthy, RS; Chu, FF; Brigelius-Flohé, R. Glutathione peroxidase-2 and selenium decreased inflammation and tumors in a mouse model of inflammation-associated carcinogenesis whereas sulforaphane effects differed with selenium supply. *Carcinogenesis* 2012,33,620–8.

[108] Ock, CY; Kim, EH; Choi, DJ; Lee, HJ; Hahm, KB; Chung, MH. 8-Hydroxy-deoxyguanosine: not mere biomarker for oxidative stress, but remedy for oxidative stress-implicated gastrointestinal diseases. *World J. Gastroenterol.* 2012,18,302–8.

[109] Ock, CY; Kim, EH; Hong, H; Hong, KS; Han, YM; Choi, KS; Hahm, KB; Chung MH. Prevention of colitis-associated colorectal cancer with 8-hydroxydeoxyguanosine. *Cancer Prev. Res.*(Phila) 2011,4,1507–1521.

[110] Yamaguchi, K; Shiozaki, K; Moriya, S; Koseki, K; Wada, T; Tateno, H; Sato, I; Asano, M; Iwakura, Y; Miyagi, T. Reduced susceptibility to colitis-associated colon carcinogenesis in mice lacking plasma membrane-associated sialidase. *PLoS One* 2012,7,e41132.

[111] Jauch, D; Martin, M; Schiechl, G; Kesselring, R; Schlitt, HJ; Geissler, EK; Fichtner-Feigl, S. Interleukin 21 controls tumour growth and tumour immunosurveillance in colitis-associated tumorigenesis in mice. *Gut* 2011,60,1678–86.

[112] D'Errico, I; Salvatore, L; Murzilli, S; Lo Sasso, G; Latorre, D; Martelli, N; Egorova, AV; Polishuck, R; Madeyski-Bengtson, K; Lelliott, C; Vidal-Puig, AJ; Seibel, P; Villani, G; Moschetta, A. Peroxisome proliferator-activated receptor-gamma coactivator 1-alpha (PGC1alpha) is a metabolic regulator of intestinal epithelial cell fate. *Proc. Natl. Acad. Sci. USA* 2011,108,6603–8.

[113] Tanaka, T; Kohno, H; Yoshitani, S; Takashima, S; Okumura, A; Murakami, A; Hosokawa, M. Ligands for peroxisome proliferator-activated receptors alpha and gamma inhibit chemically induced colitis and formation of aberrant crypt foci in rats. *Cancer Res.* 2001,61,2424–8.

[114] Wang, D; DuBois, RN. Peroxisome proliferator-activated receptors in chronic inflammation and colorectal cancer. *Gastroenterol. Clin. North* Am 2010,39,697–707.

[115] Takahashi, N; Okumura, T; Motomura, W; Fujimoto, Y; Kawabata, I; Kohgo, Y. Activation of PPARgamma inhibits cell growth and induces apoptosis in human gastric cancer cells. *FEBS Lett.* 1999,455,135–9.

[116] Kohno, H; Yoshitani, S; Takashima, S; Okumura, A; Hosokawa, M; Yamaguchi, N; Tanaka, T. Troglitazone, a ligands for peroxisome proliferator-activated receptor gamma, inhibits chemically-induced aberrant crypt foci in rats. *Jpn J. Cancer Res.* 2001,92,396–403.

[117] Su, W; Necela, BM; Fujiwara, K; Kurakata, S; Murray, NR; Fields, AP; Thompson, EA. The high affinity peroxisome proliferator-activated receptor-gamma agonist RS5444 inhibits both initiation and progression of colon tumors in azoxymethanetreated miceInt. *J. Cancer* 2008, 123, 991–7.

[118] Osawa, E; Nakajima, A; Wada, K; Ishimine, S; Fujisawa, N; Kawamori, T; Matsuhashi, N; Kadowaki T; Ochiai, M; Sekihara, H; Nakagama, H. Peroxisome proliferator-activated receptor gamma ligands suppress colon carcinogenesis induced by azoxymethane in mice. *Gastroenterology* 2003,124,361–7.

[119] Chumanevich, AA; Poudyal, D; Cui, X; Davis, T; Wood, PA; Smith, CD; Hofseth, LJ. Suppression of colitis-driven colon cancer in mice by a novel small molecule inhibitor of sphingosine kinase. *Carcinogenesis* 2010,31,1787–93.

[120] Suzuki, S; Sakamoto, S; Mitamura, T; Sassa, S; Kudo, H; Yamashita, Y. Preventive effects of sulphasalazine on colorectal carcinogenesis in mice with ulcerative colitis. *In Vivo* 2000,14,463–6.

[121] Clapper, ML; Gary, MA; Coudry, RA; Litwin, S; Chang, WC; Devarajan, K; Lubet, RA; Cooper, HS. 5-aminosalicylic acid inhibits colitis-associated colorectal dysplasias in the mouse model of azoxymethane/dextran sulfate sodium-induced colitis. *Inflamm Bowel Dis.* 2008,14,1341–7.
[122] Kohno, H; Suzuki, R; Yasui, Y; Miyamoto, S; Wakabayashi, K; Tanaka, T. Ursodeoxycholic acid versus sulfasalazine in colitis-related colon carcinogenesis in mice. *Clin. Cancer Res.* 2007,13,2519–25.
[123] Stolfi, C; Sarra, M; Caruso, R; Fantini, MC; Fina, D; Pellegrini, R; Palmieri, G; Macdonald, TT; Pallone, F; Monteleone, G. Inhibition of colon carcinogenesis by 2-methoxy-5-amino-N-hydroxybenzamide, a novel derivative of mesalamine. *Gastroenterology* 2010,138,221–30.
[124] Kohno, H; Suzuki, R; Sugie, S; Tanaka, T. Suppression of colitis-related mouse colon carcinogenesis by a COX-2 inhibitor and PPAR ligands. *BMC Cancer* 2005,5,46.
[125] Glauben, R; Batra, A; Stroh, T; Erben, U; Fedke, I; Lehr, HA; Leoni, F; Mascagni, P; Dinarello, CA; Zeitz, M; Siegmund, B. Histone deacetylases: novel targets for prevention of colitis-associated cancer in mice. *Gut* 2008,57,613–22.

In: Animal Models in Cancer Research …
Editor: Sean A. Murray

ISBN: 978-1-62417-587-9

Chapter II

Large Animal Models of Human Cardiovascular Disease

Naritatsu Saito*[1]*, and Fumiaki Ikeno*[2]
[1]Cardiovascular Medicine, Kyoto University、Kyoto, Japan
[2]Cardiovascular Medicine, Stanford University, Stanford, California, US

Abstract

In most countries, cardiovascular disease is one of the leading causes of death. The treatment and management of cardiovascular disease has advanced over the past 2 decades, largely due to the use of experimental animal models. Although a large amount of information can be generated with the use of experimental animal models, non-human animal models cannot fully replicate the complexity of human pathological conditions. Thus, a deeper understanding of the differences and similarities between humans and each animal model is important in preclinical research. Small animal models provide insight into the molecular and cellular basis of cardiovascular biology, but significant differences exist with regard to cardiovascular characteristics between small animal models and humans. Large animal models which simulate human cardiovascular physiology, anatomy and function are also crucial to develop clinical therapies and interventions. Here, we will mainly focus on the large animal models of cardiovascular disease, including coronary artery disease, heart failure, peripheral artery disease and structural heart disease.

Introduction

Cardiovascular diseases are the leading cause of death and morbidity in most developed countries. The treatment and management of cardiovascular disease have advanced drama-

* Corresponding Author: Fumiaki Ikeno, MD, 300 Pasteur Drive, FALK Cardiovascular research center, Stanford, CA 94305-5406, USA, P: +1-650-724-1579, E-mail: fikeno@stanford.edu.

tically over the past 2 decades, largely dependent on research findings from animal models. Numerous cardiovascular animal models have been developed in many species. Animal models of cardiovascular disease have yielded invaluable information into human cardiovascular disease, and have also provided a test bed for pharmacological, surgical, and catheter-based interventional treatments. However, non-human animal models cannot fully replicate the complexity of human pathological conditions.

Thus, the investigator should understand the differences and similarities between humans and each animal model. Small animal models are more applicable to research work compared to large animal models due to their low cost and convenience in handling.

However, significant differences exist with regard to cardiovascular characteristics between small animal models and humans. Large animal models approximating human anatomy, function, and physiology are indispensable when translating basic scientific discoveries and technologies into clinical applications. This chapter mainly focuses on the large animal models of cardiovascular disease, including coronary artery disease, heart failure, peripheral artery disease and structural heart disease.

1. Animal Models of Coronary Artery Disease

Coronary artery disease represents a very heterogeneous group of diseases including myocardial infarction, transient or chronic myocardial ischemia, heart failure and death. In this section, the animal model of each phenotype of coronary artery disease is described.

1.1. Myocardial Infarction

Swine are superior large animal models for studies of myocardial infarction because the shapes of swine coronary arteries are comparable to those of the human coronary artery, whereas canines have an extensive collateral coronary circulation, making consistent degrees of myocardial injury difficult, potentially altering the post myocardial infarction course [1]. Myocardial infarction in the swine model can be achieved by fully blocking or partially narrowing the coronary artery, which can be achieved by a surgical procedure or catheter intervention.

Surgical ligation of the coronary arteries with thoracotomy to induce myocardial infarction has been used for more than half a century [2–8]. Ligation of the left anterior descending artery to create an anterior wall infarction is most frequently used. Permanent ligation of the left anterior descending artery causes irreversible damage to the left ventricle, which is stable and reproducible. The subsequent removal of the occlusion can create an ischemia-reperfusion model, which is also applied in studies on myocardial infarction therapy using techniques such as cell implantation [6], administration of cytokines, and gene therapy [7]. The main advantage of surgical ligation is the creation of a reproducible and stable myocardial infarction. This approach also provides easy access to the heart for coronary ligation as well as assessment of tissue metabolic parameters during and after the ligation. One disadvantage of this model is the requirement for thoracotomy, which relates to complications such as delayed recovery from anesthesia, infection, and increased mortality.

Furthermore, opening the chest and pericardium are reported to influence the pattern of left ventricular remodeling after myocardial infarction in the chronic model [8]. Thoracotomy also influences imaging properties of the animals. Magnetic resonance image quality is degraded in animal models of myocardial infarction induced by thoracotomy due to the presence of increased amounts of air in tissue layers [9].

Less invasive catheter-based techniques are also widely used to create myocardial infarction. Cardiac catheterization and coronary intervention in swine have many similarities to those in humans. For skilled interventional cardiologists, performing cardiac catheterization in swine is not difficult.

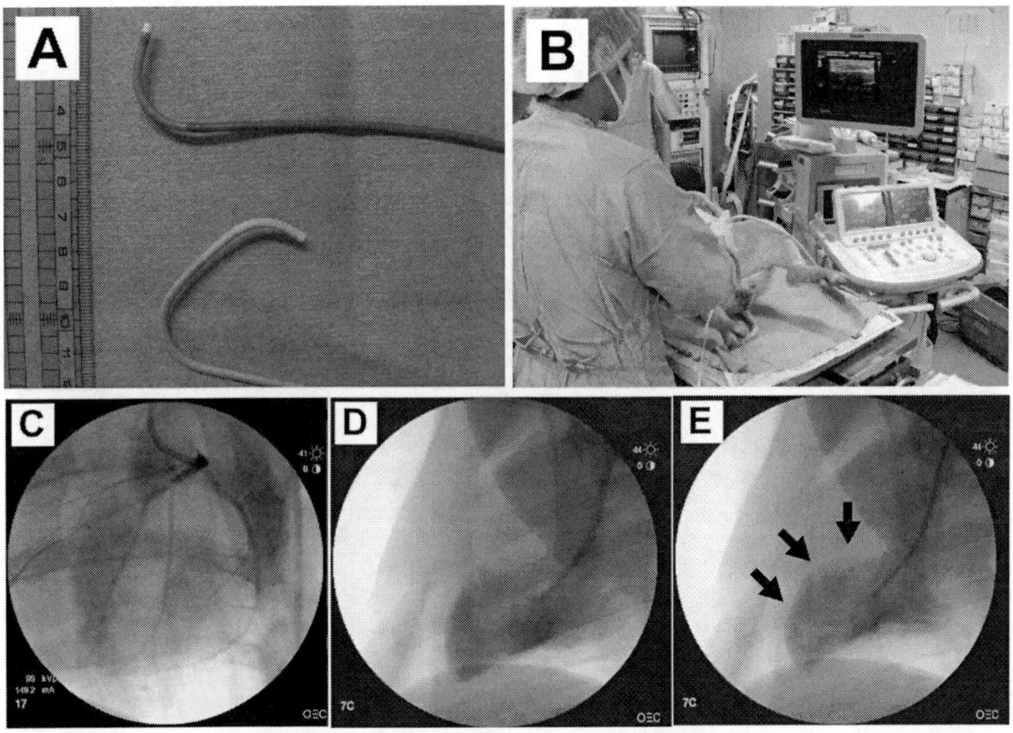

Figure 1. A technique for creating a catheter-based coronary occlusion model in swine. A, A 7Fr Judkins left 4.0 guide catheter is usually applied when approaching from the carotid artery. A 7Fr Hockey Stick guide catheter is used when approaching from the femoral artery. B, Sheath introduction is usually conducted percutaneously under echo guidance in the animal laboratory in Kyoto University. In this case, the introduction sheath is placed in the femoral artery. C, The left coronary artery is engaged by the Hockey Stick guide catheter, and the middle portion of the left anterior descending artery is occluded with a 3.0 mm balloon catheter. D, Post infarction left ventriculography in diastole. E, Post infarction left ventriculography in systole showing decreased wall motion in the anterior wall [arrows], which indicates that the creation of myocardial infarction is successful.

Injection of thrombogenic materials such as microcoils or thrombin-fibrinogen mixtures into the coronary artery can be applied to create myocardial infarction in an animal model. However, controlling the duration and location of coronary occlusion is not possible with this approach. Currently, an injection or placement of foreign bodies into the coronary artery is not frequently used for creating myocardial infarction models. This technique is applied more often in a coronary chronic total occlusion model or heart failure model [10]. Placement of a balloon catheter in the coronary artery and inflation of the balloon to achieve occlusion avoids thoracotomy and allows control of the location and time of occlusion. Several articles have described that balloon occlusion of the left anterior descending artery can be successfully conducted in swine to create reperfused or occlusive myocardial infarction [9,11–13]. Figure 1 depicts the technique for creating the catheter-based coronary occlusion model in swine. The technique is simpler and more convenient compared to surgical ligation. The consecutive changes of cardiac function are considered solely due to ischemia, rendering results obtained with this model more easily interpretable.

This model has another advantage in magnetic resonance image studies because susceptibility artifacts that arise in open-chest models can be avoided.

1.2. Chronic Ischemia and Ischemic Cardiomyopathy

An animal model of chronic coronary stenosis resulting in hibernating myocardium and ischemic cardiomyopathy is also important in preclinical studies for small molecule delivery, gene transfer and stem cell therapy. Several studies have described various methods to induce ischemic cardiomyopathy in large animal models [14]. Implantation of the ameroid constrictor in the coronary artery causes complete or partial occlusion of the coronary artery. The main disadvantage of the ameroid constrictor model is the high mortality rate when implanting it in the left anterior descending artery [14].

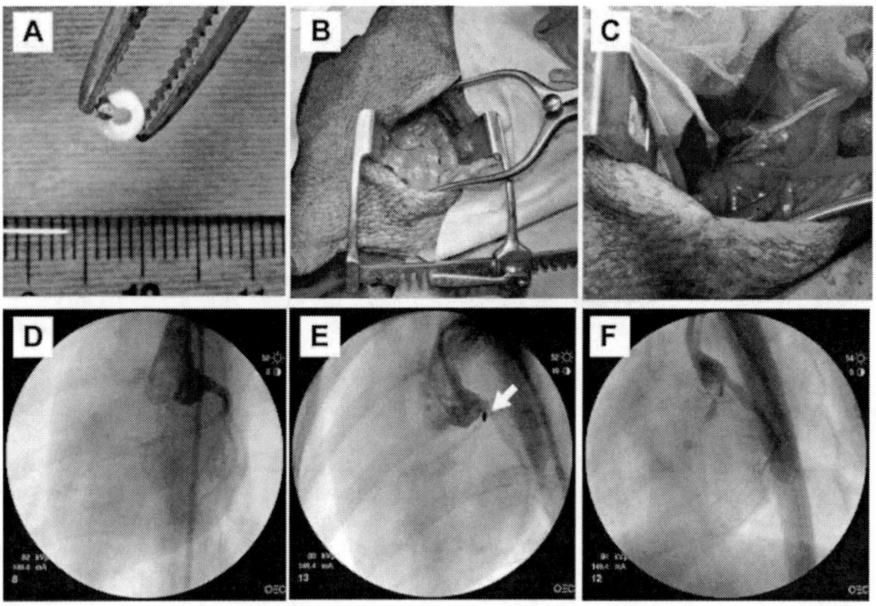

Figure 2. A technique to induce ischemic cardiomyopathy in the swine model. A, A plastic occluder with a fixed diameter of 1.0 mm fitted with an 18-gauge copper wire. B, Surgical access is achieved through the third left intercostal space. C, The plastic occluder is deployed around the proximal segment of the left anterior descending coronary artery and fixed loosely with cotton umbilical tape. D, Left coronary angiography before occluder deployment without any coronary stenosis.E, Left coronary angiography just after occluder deployment showing a stenosis in the proximal left anterior descending coronary artery. Arrow indicates copper wire. F, Left coronary angiography at 1 month follow-up showing total occlusion of the proximal left anterior descending coronary artery with birding ?bridging collaterals.

Thus, the ameroid constrictor is mainly applied to the left circumflex to avoid animal death. Because the left circumflex artery supplies smaller areas of the myocardium compared to other coronary arteries, the depression of cardiac function remains small. Thus, when considering an animal model with severe cardiac dysfunction, the ameroid constrictor model is not suitable. Ishikawa and colleagues have described a more sophisticated method to induce progressive coronary artery stenosis, utilizing a plastic occluder with a fixed diameter of 1.0 mm, fitted with an 18-gauge copper wire which is placed around the proximal left anterior descending artery in swine [15,16]. In this model, chronic ischemia in the proximal left anterior descending artery is induced with a low mortality rate of less than 30%[15]. Figure 2 briefly describes their method.

1.3. Coronary Artery Stenosis

When focusing on the coronary artery itself, an animal model of chronic coronary ischemia can be described as an animal model of coronary stenosis. The animal model of coronary artery stenosis is important for cardiovascular device testing, physician training, development of coronary imaging technologies and for the study of coronary blood flow and flow reserve. Swine are the most suitable animals for fulfilling these purposes. Several methods have been proposed to create reproducible coronary artery stenosis in swine. Simple dilatation of a normal swine coronary artery with an oversized balloon creates a slit-like medial rupture which heals over the course of 2 to 4 weeks, rarely resulting in a significant coronary stenosis. Oversized stenting creates a more exuberant healing response that sometimes, but not always, results in late luminal narrowing [17]. A fundamental disadvantage of the stent restenosis model is that the stent itself is a foreign body which can produce artifact in imaging studies such as computed tomography, magnetic resonance imaging and intravascular ultrasound. This model is not suitable to evaluate the performance of the novel stent system because the previously implanted stent is disturbed. Several groups have reported that the swine heat injury model is more reliable [18,19]. Suzuki and colleagues described that coronary artery stenoses were consistently developed at 4 weeks after thermal balloon angioplasty at a high temperature of 80°C for 80 seconds [18]. Using this technique, the heat injury model can be applicable for imaging studies and the evaluation of novel stent systems.

1.4. Chronic Total Occlusion

Chronic total occlusion is the complete blockage of the coronary artery. Special techniques and dedicated devices are often required for the treatment of chronic total occlusion. Technically, chronic total occlusion is considered the final challenge in interventional cardiology.

A large animal model of chronic total occlusion closely mimicking human chronic total occlusion would facilitate the development of novel devices and techniques to enhance procedural success rates. Spontaneous plaque rupture and subsequent coronary occlusion do not usually occur in any animal models. Initial animal models relied on surgically placed ameroid constrictors which cause gradual coronary occlusion by external compression [14]. However, this method would not be appropriate for the evaluation of novel chronic total occlusion devices.

The percutaneous implantation of a copper stent was also examined [19,20]. Copper stents are highly immunogenic and can cause inflammatory reactions subsequently resulting in coronary occlusion. Other percutaneous approaches include thrombin injection [21], thermal injury [18,19], polymer-coated stent implantation [22] and the deployment of a microporous poly L-lactic acid polymer [23], all of which cause inflammatory reactions in the coronary artery and coronary occlusions. The histology of these inflammatory agent implant-tations showed mature fibrous tissue, neointimal proliferation, multiple small intraluminal vascular channels and disruption of internal elastic lamina, which are characteristics of human chronic total occlusions. However, none of them showed calcification, which is also an important characteristic of human chronic total occlusions. There are 2 methods for creating swine calcified coronary total occlusions. One method applies crushed swine bone chips with an absorbable sponge [24] and another method applies anapatite-coated absorbable sponge [10]. In both methods, calcified chronic total occlusions were reproducibly created by implanting these materials. The main disadvantage of these methods is a high mortality of 30 to 40%.

This is because the coronary arteries are abruptly occluded and inevitably cause myocardial infarction. These models can reproduce characteristics of human coronary chronic total occlusion including microvascular channels and microcalcifications, which makes the model especially valuable for the investigation of novel devices, pharmacological investigation, and physician training.

1.5. Animal Models for the Evaluation of Drug Eluting Stents

Although bare metal stent implantation (BMS) can prevent elastic vascular recoil and constrictive arterial remodeling, local deep vascular injury induces more neointimal hyperplasia than balloon angioplasty alone, leading to an in-stent restenosis in approximately 20% of patients [25]. Pivotal randomized clinical trials have shown that first generation drug-eluting stents (DES) with anti-proliferative agents markedly reduced restenosis [26,27]. However, late and very late stent thrombosis in DES patients has emerged as a major concern [28]. Pathological studies in patients with DES thrombosis demonstrated delayed arterial healing, characterized by persistent fibrin deposition and poor endothelialization of the stent struts [29]. Recently, another pathological study showed that neoatherosclerosis is frequently observed in DES-covered segments which occur earlier compared with BMS-covered segments [30]. This observation indicates that neoatherosclerosis could be accelerated after DES implantation and could be related to very late thrombotic events. These study findings suggest that DES-tissue interactions are so complex that a multidisciplinary approach is required for preclinical study to predict clinical safety and efficacy; the evaluation of operational performance, structural integrity and long-term biocompatibility using appropriate animal models are mandatory prior to investigation in patients.

Several animal models are proposed for the evaluation of DES. Rabbit iliac arteries and swine coronary arteries are the two most widely used animal arteries in assessing DES safety and possibly efficacy. An updated consensus recommendation for preclinical evaluation of

DES recommends that the stent should be appropriately sized (stent: vessel ratio between 1.1 and 1.0) and implanted into arteries without prior injury in both models [31], while using a higher stent/artery ratio could induce severe arterial injury and considerable stenosis [32]. Several sampling time points are also recommended [31]. Clinical and histopathologic data should be obtained at an early time point of 3 to 7 days to evaluate subacute thrombosis risk by comparing a mean thrombus/neointimal area for DES and BMS controls. Short-term endpoints are required when endothelialization rates are the objective of the study: less than 14 days for swine coronary arteries and 28 days for rabbit iliac arteries. The 28 day time point is the most important to quantitate neointimal hyperplasia. Two or more late time points (e.g. 180 and 360 days) are also recommended to examine the longterm effects of DES, specifically neointimal hyperplasia, arterial healing, residual fibrin deposition, calcification, inflammation, granuloma formation and qualitative vascular cellularity. The 3 months time point is usually acceptable for initiating investigational device exemption clinical trials if no adverse findings are detected at this time point, and if vascular responses are no worse than earlier time points. Each animal model has its own advantages and disadvantages. Rabbits are small, easy to handle, relatively inexpensive and do not gain excessive body weight within a short time period when compared to swine. Furthermore, the rabbit iliac artery model is considered more suitable to evaluate endothelialization of DES because the processes of healing are slower compared to the swine coronary artery model. However, one limitation is that foam cells are commonly found in this model, whereas they are rare in human restenoticneointima. The advantages and disadvantages of the 2 preclinical animal models are listed in Table 1.

The investigators should understand the differences and advantages of each model and choose the appropriate one for the hypothesis being examined.

Table 1. Advantages and disadvantages of the rabbit iliac arteries model compared with the swine coronary arteries model for the evaluation of drug- eluting stents

	Rabbit Iliac Arteries	Pig Coronary Arteries
Cost	Inexpensive	Expensive
Feeding, Housing, Handling	Easy	Difficult
Body Weight Change	Minimum	Large
Endothelialization	Slow	Fast
Inflammation	Not Extensive	Extensive
Other Advantages	Provides additional data, especially regarding endothelialization	Responds similar to human coronary arteries
Other Disadvantages	Vessels are smaller and the reaction to injury is less defined	Injury models vary more widely in biologic response, thus affecting reliability and reproducibility of the evaluation

2. Animal Models of Heart Failure

Heart failure is a clinical syndrome with primary symptoms including dyspnea, fatigue, exercise intolerance, and retention of fluid in the lungs and peripheral tissue. Heart failure results from multiple origins and diverse etiologies and relates to poor outcomes, independent of specific courses. Although meaningful insight into the molecular and cellular basis of cardiovascular biology can be provided from small animal models, significant differences exist with regard to cardiac characteristics such as heart size, contractility, heart rate, oxygen consumption, adrenergic receptor ratios and response to loss of regulatory proteins. Larger animal models of heart failure, which more closely simulate human physiology, are also essential. In this section, several methods to induce heart failure in large animals are described. The readers should note that most models use young healthy animals, whereas heart failure in humans is a disease of the elderly. Moreover, heart failure in humans is often associated with atherosclerosis, but the development of atherosclerosis is unusual in most large animals.

2.1. Ischemia

Heart failure is frequently precipitated by myocardial ischemia or infarction. A common phenotype of myocardial ischemia is heart failure. Various methods to induce myocardial ischemia or infarction including surgical ligation of the coronary artery, balloon occlusion, the application of an ameroid constrictor and others have already been described in the previous section. All these animal models employed occlusion or narrowing of the epicardial large coronary arteries. In this section, myocardial ischemia induced by microembolization of the coronary arteries is described.

Coronary microembolization has been used extensively to create myocardial ischemia and subsequent heart failure in various large animal species [33–35]. Multiple sequential intracoronary embolizations with microspheresfrom70 to 100 μm in diameter produce numerous micro-infarcts in the myocardium which are caused by mechanical occlusion of the coronary arterioles with microvascular vasoconstriction. Although micro-infarction would not necessarily result in transmural ischemia or necrosis, the cumulative effect of repeated micro-infarctions would deteriorate cardiac and endothelial function, finally resulting in heart failure. A canine was employed as the animal model in the initial article described by Sabah and colleagues [34]. In the article, coronary embolizations into the left anterior descending or circumflex artery were conducted using polystyrene latex microspheres of 77 to 102 μm in diameter in a closed chest model. With 3 to 9embolizations performed 1 to 3 weeks apart, left ventricular function was significantly altered. Embolization were discontinued when the LV ejection fraction became less than 35%. An important feature of the microembolization model of heart failure is the observation of a lack of recovery of left ventricular function after discontinuation of the embolizations. Partial recovery of left ventricular function after acute coronary occlusion has been described in canines, accounted for by the presence of substantial collateral circulation. In the microembolization model of heart failure, sequential multiple embolization gradually exhausts the compensatory mechanisms available to the myocardium. Thus, myocardial ischemia induced by microembolization is considered an irreversible model of heart failure. A limitation of the embolization model is that the exact location and length of the coronary artery occlusion is unknown. Another disadvantage is that the creation of the model requires serial catheter interventions that are time consuming. However, the low risk of infection and inflammatory complications is a distinct advantage of the model as coronary arteryembolizations are inducible percutaneously and do not require surgical intervention such as thoracotomy.

2.2. Volume Overload

Acute volume overload with isotonic fluids or colloids has long been used to reproduce the hemodynamic condition of congestion in chronic heart failure [36]. Toyoda and colleagues described that a central venous infusion of 10 mg/kg of 4.5% albumin solution for 5 minutes can cause heart failure in beagles. This method can be used alone, but is more commonly applied with another model of heart failure. Volume overload will enhance the hemodynamic changes induced by the model of heart failure [37,38]. The method is considered effective for evaluating diastolic dysfunction after induction of heart failure.

Other approaches to induce a volume overload state are the creation of an arteriovenous fistula and induction of mitral regurgitation [39,40]. Bolotin and colleagues described that the creation of an arteriovenous fistula between the carotid artery and jugular vein in gout induced a marked increase of cardiac output and left ventricle end-diastolic diameter at 8 weeks after the procedure [39]. Another study described that a combination of surgical creation of an arteriovenous fistula and weekly intravenous doxorubicin injections resulted in heart failure more effectively [41]. A higher dose of doxorubicin was associated with more pronounced left ventricular dysfunction and was associated with clinical symptoms of heart failure.

Induction of mitral regurgitation is also commonly applied to induce volume overload. Mitral regurgitation in a large animal model can be created using a percutaneous method [37,42]. Briefly, an introducer sheath is placed into the left ventricle through the carotid artery under fluoroscopic guidance. Flexible rat-tooth forceps are inserted through the introducer sheath. Then, the chordae tendineae of the mitral valve apparatus are ruptured by the forceps. This percutaneous method is reported to be applicable to canines and swine. Mitral regurgitation has a number of underlying etiologies. Various methods for creating mitral regurgitation in large animal models have been reported. The mechanism of functional or ischemic mitral regurgitation, which is a common sequel to various cardiomyopathies, has been extensively studied by using various large animal models. These animal models of mitral regurgitation are described in another section.

2.3. Pressure Overload

Another model of heart failure in large animals is pressure overload of the left ventricle. Pressure overload of the left ventricle causes a compensatory increase in left ventricular mass, which affects left ventricular stiffness and reduces relaxation, ultimately resulting in heart failure. The model is considered most suitable for studying diastolic dysfunction which is an important factor in the development of heart failure [43]. Chien and colleagues described a surgical method to induce pressure overload of the left ventricle by creating supravalvular aortic stenosis with narrowing of the aorta above the aortic valve in canines [44]. In brief, the ascending aorta was dissected free from the pulmonary artery. The ascending aorta was then encircled by a 1.5 to 2 cm wide, 6 to 7 cm long dacron patch. A J-shaped clamp was applied to the ascending aorta at the dacron patch. Two layers of continuous mattress suture were placed adjacent to the clamp, plicating the aortic diameter by about 50%. An additional one or two deep mattress sutures were placed below the running mattress sutures to increase the stenosis and to obtain the aimed gradient of 50 to 60 mmHg. A more simple and sophisticated method for creating an ovine pressure overload model was developed by Moorjani and colleagues [45]. A variable constriction device, which consisted of a Gore-Tex cuff enclosing the balloon cuff of a Foley catheter, was surgically passed around the ascending aorta just proximal to the origin of the innominate artery. Aimed transcoarctation pressure gradient was gained by inflating the balloon. This method can be applicable to other animals. Yarbrough and colleagues described a similar method to induce left ventricular pressure overload in swine [46]. These models have made it possible to induce progressive increase of afterload on the left ventricle which results in left ventricular hypertrophy. The readers should note that these models produce marked left ventricular hypertrophy, but do not reproduce neurohormonal activation or left ventricular systolic dysfunction [47]. The banding method is also applicable to induce right heart ventricular hypertrophy. The pulmonary artery constriction device is employed to induce pressure overload of the right ventricle [48]. Another model of pressure overload in the right ventricle results from pulmonary hypertension [49,50]. Monocrotaline, which is a pyrrolizidine alkaloid found in the plant species Crotalaria spectabilis, has been used to induce pulmonary hypertension in large animals. Monocrotaline injections into the right atrium cause pulmonary vascular syndrome characterized by proliferative pulmonary vasculitis, pulmonary hypertension and corpulmonale.

Induction of systemic hypertension can also cause pressure overload of the left ventricle. A canine model of systemic hypertension produced by wrapping 1 kidney in silk and subsequently performing contralateral nephrectomy has been reported [51]. Recently, several variants of this model have been described in large animal models [52].

2.4. Rapid Pacing

Sustained rapid pacing of the heart has been used to produce a simple, reliable and reversible model of heart failure in different animal species. This includes rabbits, canines, swine, and sheep [53]. The right ventricle or atrium is paced at 200 to 400 beats per minute which produces severe biventricular systolic dysfunction, resulting in congestive heart failure at 3 to 5 weeks. Hemodynamic changes occur soon after rapid pacing with continued deterioration of ventricular function up to 3 to 5 weeks. After stopping the rapid pacing, systolic dysfunction shows significant recovery with subsequent normalization in 1 to 2 weeks. Diastolic dysfunction is also considered and persists for longer than systolic dysfunction. The rapid pacing model closely replicates the mechanical, structural, neurohormonal and myocyte functional alterations of dilated cardiomyopathy in humans and has been used to test pharmacological and gene therapies [53–55].

2.5. Toxins

Several drugs, including ergonovine, isoproterenol and doxorubicin are used to induce heart failure in various animal species [56–59]. Ergonovine and isoproterenol are mainly used for small animals. In contrast, doxorubicin is often employed for large animals. Dose-related doxorubicin cardiac toxicity has already been documented in several animal species with different modes of application. Van Vleet and colleagues employed intravenous administration of doxorubicin with significantly higher doses in swine [56]. However, severe side effects affecting nearly all organs caused by the high doxorubicin doses were described in the article. Therefore, systemic administration of doxorubicin is not recommended for ethical reasons. Toyoda and colleagues performed a catheterization of the left main coronary and applied a low-dose [0.7 mg/kg] doxorubicin infusion into the left main coronary artery [58]. Infusions were repeated weekly for 5 weeks. The left ventricular function was significantly decreased at 3 months. Intracoronary injection allows delivery of doxorubicin at a smaller dose to induce heart failure without systemic toxicity. In contrast, a disadvantage of the model is that it requires repeated punctures of the femoral artery each week, which is time consuming and becomes more and more difficult with increasing numbers of punctures. Christiansen and colleagues described a method that omits the repetitive punctures and catheterizations, in which an intracoronary catheter was implanted directly into the left main stem in swine and connected to a percutaneous access port that was used for repetitive injections of doxorubicin [59].

3. Animal Models of Peripheral Artery Disease

Atherosclerosis is the leading cause of morbidity and mortality in most developed countries. Peripheral artery occlusive disease is a phenotype of atherosclerosis. Several preclinical models of peripheral artery disease have been proposed. In this section, the large animal model of peripheral artery disease will be discussed.

3.1. Thrombin Injection

In the 1950s, Longland proposed a method to establish an animal model of chronic hindlimb ischemia by injecting thrombin and sclerosant into the femoral artery of rabbits [60,61]. Although the model was associated with a high incidence of mortality, it provided the conceptual framework for future chronic lower-extremity ischemia models. To date, several modifications have been introduced to the technique. Labs and colleagues described a method to develop a canine model of thrombotic iliac artery occlusion [62]. The iliac artery was surgically isolated, and spring loaded vascular clips were then placed on the proximal and distal aspect of the iliac artery. Then, iliac artery thrombosis was induced by the injection of approximately 400 units of bovine thrombin. The vascular clips were removed 3 to 9 days after the thrombin injection. A stable thrombus of known age and organization was reproducibly obtained in this model. This model is recommended for studies of thrombotic vascular occlusive disease, especially when quantification of thrombus volume is desirable.

3.2. Surgical Ligation

Surgical ligation of the lower extremity inflow vessels has also been employed in an attempt to create states of hindlimb ischemia in animals. The reader should note that species to species variations of collateral blood flow exist just like the coronary circulation; canines have richer lower-extremity collateral pathways when compared to swine [60]. A swine femoral artery ligation model with reductions in resting ischemic limb blood pressure and blood flow by internal flow probe lasting 2 weeks has been described [63]. The swine ligation model was considered suitable for the evaluation of arteriogenic effects of growth factors or genes by assessing the growth of collateral arteries.

3.3. Mechanical Injury Induced Neointimal Hyperplasia

Restenosis after successful endovascular interventions remains a major limitation to long term therapeutic success in the treatment of peripheral artery disease [64].

Therapeutic modalities that may have the potential to prevent neointimal hyperplasia inevitably need to be tested in large animal models before their human clinical use. However, mechanical injuries by over-distension with an oversized balloon dilatation induce subtle neointimal hyperplasia in swine iliac arteries [65]. The endovascular injury model that is capable of inducing significant neointima in pig iliac arteries within 4 weeks is an oversized metallic stent injury [66].

However, the stent restenosis model is often inappropriate because the stent itself is a foreign body. Moreover, the stent can produce artifacts in imaging studies, and can hamper the evaluation of a novel stent system. Interestingly, peripheral arteries are less prone to develop significant neointimal hyperplasia and subsequent restenosis than coronary arteries in the swine model [67], which makes the stent restenosis model in the swine iliac artery less valuable in preclinical studies. Houbballah and colleagues described a novel method to induce accelerated neointimal hyperplasia in swine iliac arteries [65]. Arterial wall disruption was achieved by pulling back an isometric cutting balloon followed by stretching with a compliant Fogarty Balloon. Significant neointimal hyperplasia comparable to the stent restenosis model was observed at 2 weeks after the procedure. This model is useful to test novel therapies aimed at limiting neointimal hyperplasia in large diameter peripheral arteries.

4. Animal Models of Structural Heart Disease

Structural heart disease is a new term which refers to congenital heart disease and acquired heart disease involving structural and functional abnormalities of heart valves, cardiac chambers and the proximal great vessels [68]. Structural heart disease interventions have emerged as a new field in interventional cardiology within the last decade. The advancement of structural heart disease interventions was largely due to findings of animal experiments. However, most of the novel therapeutic devices for structural heart disease were tested using healthy animals. Large animal models of structural heart disease are poorly available, except for animal models of ischemic mitral regurgitation. In this section, several animal models of ischemic mitral regurgitation are described.

4.1. Ischemic Mitral Regurgitation

Ischemic mitral regurgitation, also referred to as functional mitral regurgitation, now receives increased attention. Ischemic mitral regurgitation usually occurs as a consequence of regional or global left ventricular dysfunction despite structurally normal leaflets [69]. Therefore, Ischemic mitral regurgitation is not considered as a disease of the valve but rather as a disease of the left ventricle. Ischemic mitral regurgitation is an independent risk factor for mortality in patients with heart failure and left ventricular systolic dysfunction [70]. The causes of ischemic mitral regurgitation are unclear, but the condition is associated with outward papillary muscle displacement, mitral annular dilatation and left ventricle dilatation. Interestingly, the presence and degree of mitral regurgitation are not associated with the severity of LV systolic function [71]. Clinical studies have confirmed that ischemic mitral regurgitation is more likely to occur after posteroinferior infarction than anterior myocardial infarction [72]. Another important fact is that the degree of ischemic mitral regurgitation varies dynamically with loading conditions that modulate left ventricular volume. For this reason, exercise echocardiography is considered as the gold standard for the diagnosis of ischemic mitral regurgitation [73].

The most extensively used experimental models of ischemic mitral regurgitation are the myocardial infarction and rapid ventricular pacing model. Several studies have described the feasibility of the infarction induced ischemic mitral regurgitation in large animals [74–80]. Most studies employed sheep and obtuse marginal branches for the targets of occlusions. The success rate of myocardial infarction-induced ischemic mitral regurgitation varied significantly, from 26% to 100%. In addition, this method was sometimes related to a high mortality rate [0-39%].

Another method to induce ischemic mitral regurgitation utilizes rapid pacing [81–83]. Although the rapid pacing method showed a high success rate for creating mitral regurgitation and low mortality rate, an important challenge with the rapid pacing model is that the biochemical and hemodynamic alterations revert to normal values soon after pacing is ended. Another problem is that the mechanism of mitral regurgitation in this model is different from human ischemic mitral regurgitation. Some articles reported that no obvious apical leaflet tethering was observed [81]. A combination of infarction and rapid pacing was also reported as being effective to induce ischemic mitral regurgitation [84]. Jensen and colleagues described that 50 swine were subjected to posterolateral myocardial infarction and tachycardiac stress. Thirty-six animals died [72%],of which ten animals [20%] developed ischemic mitral regurgitation. A high mortality rate and a low success rate of creating ischemic mitral regurgitation still remain as major problems with this model.

Table 2. Large animal models of ischemic mitral regurgitation

Authors [Year]	Species	# of Animals	Method	Mortality [%]	Successful creation of mitral regurgitation [%]
Otsuji, et al [2001][74]	Canine	7	Myocardial infarction	0/7 [0%]	7/7 [100%]
Tibayan, et al [2003][75]	Sheep	24	Myocardial infarction	8/24 [33%]	10/24 [42%]
Gorman, et al [2003][76]	Sheep	9	Myocardial infarction	0/7 [0%]	5/9 [56%]
Joudinaud, et al [2005][77]	Sheep	6	Myocardial infarction	1/6 [17%]	5/6 [83%]
Daimon, et al [2005][78]	Sheep	31	Myocardial infarction	12/31 [39%]	8/31 [26%]
Solis, et al [2010][79]	Sheep	14	Myocardial infarction	2/14 [14%]	10/14 [71%]
Schmitto, et al [2010][80]	Sheep	6	Myocardial infarction	1/6 [17%]	2/6 [33%]
Timek, et al [2001][81]	Sheep	9	Rapid pacing	0/9 [0%]	9/9 [100%]
Byrne, et al [2002][82]	Sheep	9	Rapid pacing	0/9 [0%]	9/9 [100%]
Kaye, et al [2003][82]	Sheep	9	Rapid pacing	0/9 [0%]	9/9 [100%]
Jensen, et al [2010][84]	Pig	50	Myocardial infarction plus rapid pacing	36/50 [72%]	10/50 [20%]

Conclusion

Various large animal models of several cardiovascular diseases are described in this chapter. The investigators need to carefully consider their choice of model. Every animal model has advantages and limitations and none of them perfectly recreates the complex pathological conditions seen in human cardiovascular disease.

Experiments in large animals are more difficult than in small animals. Large animals are generally expensive to purchase and maintain, and difficult to handle. However, large animal models provide invaluable information about human cardiovascular disease and will continue to play a crucial role in translating basic science to clinical applications for patients with cardiovascular disease.

Acknowledgment

In the preparation of this manuscript, we thank Heidi Bonneau, RN, MS, CCA for her editorial review.

References

[1] McCall FC, Telukuntla KS, Karantalis V, Suncion VY, Heldman AW, Mushtaq M, Williams AR, Hare JM. Myocardial infarction and intramyocardial injection models in swine. *Nature Protocols* [Internet]. 2012 Jul 12;7[8]:1479–1496.

[2] Gelsomino S, Lucà F, Renzulli A, Rubino AS, Romano SM, van der Veen FH, Carella R, Maessen JG, Gensini GF, Lorusso R. Increased coronary blood flow and cardiac contractile efficiency with intraaortic balloon counterpulsation in a porcine model of myocardial ischemia-reperfusion injury. *ASAIO journal [American Society for Artificial Internal Organs* : 1992] [Internet]. 2011;57[5]:375–81.

[3] JOHNS TNP, OLSON BJ. Experimental myocardial infarction. I. A method of coronary occlusion in small animals. *Annals of surgery* [Internet]. 1954 Nov;140-[5]:675–82.

[4] Kamihata H, Matsubara H, Nishiue T, Fujiyama S, Tsutsumi Y, Ozono R, Masaki H, Mori Y, Iba O, Tateishi E, Kosaki a, Shintani S, Murohara T, Imaizumi T, Iwasaka T. Implantation of bone marrow mononuclear cells into ischemic myocardium enhances collateral perfusion and regional function via side supply of angioblasts, angiogenic ligands, and cytokines. *Circulation* [Internet]. 2001 Aug 28;104[9]:1046–52.

[5] Cheng Y, Yang Y, Zhang H, Li X, Kang S, Qian H, Zhao J. No-reflow disrupts the expression and distribution of connexin 43 in a swine model. *Microvascular research* [Internet]. 2011 Nov;82[3]:404–9.

[6] Xiong Q, Hill KL, Li Q, Suntharalingam P, Mansoor A, Wang X, Jameel MN, Zhang P, Swingen C, Kaufman DS, Zhang J. A fibrin patch-based enhanced delivery of human embryonic stem cell-derived vascular cell transplantation in a porcine model of postinfarction left ventricular remodeling. *Stem cells [*Dayton, Ohio] [Internet]. 2011 Feb;29[2]:367–75.

[7] Yang Z, Chen B, Sheng Z, Zhang D, Jia E, Wang W, Ma D, Zhu T, Wang L, Li C, Wang H, Cao K, Ma W. Improvement of heart function in postinfarct heart failure swine models after hepatocyte growth factor gene transfer: comparison of low-, medium- and high-dose groups. *Molecular biology reports* [Internet]. 2010 Apr;37[4]:2075–81.

[8] Edwards R, Rakhit R. A model of closed chest regional myocardial infarction in the rabbit : a clinically relevant in vivo assay system of post-infarction remodelling. 2002;383:374–383.

[9] Krombach G a, Kinzel S, Mahnken AH, Günther RW, Buecker A. Minimally invasive close-chest method for creating reperfused or occlusive myocardial infarction in swine. I*nvestigative radiology* [Internet]. 2005 Jan;40[1]:14–8.

[10] Suzuki Y, Oyane A, Ikeno F, Lyons JK, Yeung AC. Development of animal model for calcified chronic total occlusion. *Catheterization and cardiovascular interventions : official journal of the Society for Cardiac Angiography & Interventions* [Internet]. 2009 Sep;74[3]:468–75.

[11] Peukert D, Laule M, Kaufels N, Schnorr J, Taupitz M, Hamm B, Dewey M. A minimally invasive method for induction of myocardial infarction in an animal model using tungsten spirals. *The international journal of cardiovascular imaging* [Internet]. 2009 Jun;25[5]:529–35.

[12] Suzuki M, Asano H, Tanaka H, Usuda S. Development and evaluation of a new canine myocardial infarction model using a closed-chest injection of thrombogenic material. *Japanese circulation journal* [Internet]. 1999 Nov;63[11]:900–5.

[13] Suzuki Y, Lyons JK, Yeung AC, Ikeno F. In vivo porcine model of reperfused myocardial infarction: in situ double staining to measure precise infarct area/area at risk. *Catheterization and cardiovascular interventions : official journal of the Society for Cardiac Angiography & Interventions* [Internet]. 2008 Jan;71[1]:100–7.

[14] Longhurst JC, Ordway GA, Buja LM. Evaluation of coronary native and coronary collateral pressure gradients in the conscious dog. *The American journal of cardiovascular pathology* [Internet]. 1987 Jan;1[1]:79–90.

[15] Ishikawa K, Ladage D, Takewa Y, Yaniz E, Chen J, Tilemann L, Sakata S, Badimon JJ, Hajjar RJ, Kawase Y, Sakata S, Jj B, Rj H, Development KY. Development of a preclinical model of ischemic cardiomyopathy in swine. 2011;:530–537.

[16] Ishikawa K, Ladage D, Rapti K, Fernandez-Friera L, Maria Garcia-Lopez A, Sanz J, Hajjar RJ, Kawase Y, Garcia MJ. Multimodality imaging of chronic ischemia. *Cardiology research and practice* [Internet]. 2010 Jan;2011[Figure 2]:739702.

[17] Andersen HR, Maeng M, Thorwest M, Falk E. Remodeling rather than neointimal formation explains luminal narrowing after deep vessel wall injury: insights from a porcine coronary [re]stenosis model. *Circulation* [Internet]. 1996 May 1;93[9]:1716–24.

[18] Suzuki Y, Lyons JK, Yeung AC, Ikeno F. The porcine restenosis model using thermal balloon injury: comparison with the model by coronary stenting. *The Journal of invasive cardiology* [Internet]. 2008 Mar;20[3]:142–6.

[19] Staab ME, Meeker DK, Edwards WD, Camrud AR, Jorgenson MA, Camrud LJ, Srivatsa SS, Jeong MHO, Gregoire J, Holmes DR, Schwartz RS. Reliable Models of Severe Coronary Stenosis in Porcine Coronary Arteries : Lesion Induction by High Temperature or Copper Stent. *Cardiology*. 1997;10[1]:61–69.

[20] Song W, Lee J, Kim H, Shin J, Oh D, Tio F, Wong SC, Hong MK. A new percutaneous porcine coronary model of chronic total occlusion. *The Journal of invasive cardiology* [Internet]. 2005 Sep;17[9]:452–4.

[21] Jaffe R, Leung G, Munce NR, Thind AS, Leong-Poi H, Anderson KJT, Qi X, Trogadis J, Nadler A, Shiff D, Saperia J, Lockwood J, Jacobs C, Qiang B, Teitelbaum A, Dick AJ, Sparkes JD, Butany J, Wright G a, Strauss BH. Natural history of experimental arterial chronic total occlusions. *Journal of the American College of Cardiology* [Internet]. 2009 Mar 31;53[13]:1148–58.

[22] van der Giessen WJ, Lincoff AM, Schwartz RS, van Beusekom HM, Serruys PW, Holmes DR, Ellis SG, Topol EJ. Marked inflammatory sequelae to implantation of biodegradable and nonbiodegradable polymers in porcine coronary arteries. *Circulation* [Internet]. 1996 Oct 1;94[7]:1690–7.

[23] Prosser L, Agrawal CM, Polan J, Elliott J, Adams DG, Bailey SR. Implantation of oxygen enhanced, three-dimensional microporous L-PLA polymers: a reproducible porcine model of chronic total coronary occlusion. *Catheterization and cardiovascular interventions : official journal of the Society for Cardiac Angiography & Interventions* [Internet]. 2006 Mar;67[3]:412–6.

[24] Suzuki K, Saito N, Zhang G, Conditt G, McGregor J, Flynn AM, Leahy D, Glennon P, Leon MB, Hayase M. Development of a novel calcified total occlusion model in

porcine coronary arteries. *The Journal of invasive cardiology* [Internet]. 2008 Jun;20[6]:296–301.

[25] Kimura T. Long-Term Clinical and Angiographic Follow-Up After Coronary Stent Placement in Native Coronary Arteries. *Circulation* [Internet]. 2002 Jun 17;105 [25]:2986–2991.

[26] Morice M-C, Serruys PW, Sousa JE, Fajadet J, Ban Hayashi E, Perin M, Colombo A, Schuler G, Barragan P, Guagliumi G, Molnàr F, Falotico R. A randomized comparison of a sirolimus-eluting stent with a standard stent for coronary revascularization. *The New England journal of medicine* [Internet]. 2002 Jun 6;346[23]:1773–80.

[27] Park S-J, Shim WH, Ho DS, Raizner AE, Park S-W, Hong M-K, Lee CW, Choi D, Jang Y, Lam R, Weissman NJ, Mintz GS. A paclitaxel-eluting stent for the prevention of coronary restenosis. *The New England journal of medicine* [Internet]. 2003 Apr 17;348[16]:1537–45.

[28] McFadden EP, Stabile E, Regar E, Cheneau E, Ong ATL, Kinnaird T, Suddath WO, Weissman NJ, Torguson R, Kent KM, Pichard AD, Satler LF, Waksman R, Serruys PW. Late thrombosis in drug-eluting coronary stents after discontinuation of antiplatelet therapy. *Lancet* [Internet]. 2004;364[9444]:1519–21.

[29] Joner M, Finn AV, Farb A, Mont EK, Kolodgie FD, Ladich E, Kutys R, Skorija K, Gold HK, Virmani R. Pathology of drug-eluting stents in humans: delayed healing and late thrombotic risk. *Journal of the American College of Cardiology* [Internet]. 2006 Jul 4;48[1]:193–202.

[30] Nakazawa G, Otsuka F, Nakano M, Vorpahl M, Yazdani SK, Ladich E, Kolodgie FD, Finn AV, Virmani R. The pathology of neoatherosclerosis in human coronary implants bare-metal and drug-eluting stents. *Journal of the American College of Cardiology* [Internet]. 2011 Mar 15;57[11]:1314–22.

[31] Schwartz RS, Edelman E, Virmani R, Carter A, Granada JF, Kaluza GL, Chronos N a F, Robinson K a, Waksman R, Weinberger J, Wilson GJ, Wilensky RL. Drug-eluting stents in preclinical studies: updated consensus recommendations for preclinical evaluation. Circulation. *Cardiovascular interventions* [Internet]. 2008 Oct;1[2]:143–53.

[32] Suzuki Y, Yeung AC, Ikeno F. The representative porcine model for human cardiovascular disease. *Journal of biomedicine & biotechnology* [Internet]. 2011 Jan;2011:195483.

[33] Breuckmann F, Nassenstein K, Bucher C, Konietzka I, Kaiser G, Konorza T, Naber C, Skyschally A, Gres P, Heusch G, Erbel R, Barkhausen J. Systematic analysis of functional and structural changes after coronary microembolization: a cardiac magnetic resonance imaging study. *JACC. Cardiovascular imaging* [Internet]. 2009 Feb;2[2]:121–30.

[34] Sabbah HN, Stein PD, Kono T, Gheorghiade M, Levine TB, Jafri S, Hawkins ET, Goldstein S. A canine model of chronic heart failure produced by multiple sequential coronary microembolizations. *The American journal of physiology* [Internet]. 1991 Apr;260[4 Pt 2]:H1379–84.

[35] Huang Y, Hunyor SN, Jiang L, Kawaguchi O, Shirota K, Ikeda Y, Yuasa T, Gallagher G, Zeng B, Zheng X. Remodeling of the chronic severely failing ischemic sheep heart after coronary microembolization: functional, energetic, structural, and cellular responses. American journal of physiology. *Heart and circulatory physiology* [Internet]. 2004 Jun;286[6]:H2141–50.

[36] Toyoda Y, Okada M, Kashem MA, Mukai T. Effects of cardiomyoplasty on right ventricular filling during volume loading. *The Annals of thoracic surgery* [Internet]. 1998 Jun;65[6]:1676–9.

[37] Kawase Y, Ly HQ, Prunier F, Lebeche D, Shi Y, Jin H, Hadri L, Yoneyama R, Hoshino K, Takewa Y, Sakata S, Peluso R, Zsebo K, Gwathmey JK, Tardif J-C, Tanguay J-F, Hajjar RJ. Reversal of cardiac dysfunction after long-term expression of SERCA2a by gene transfer in a pre-clinical model of heart failure. *Journal of the American College of Cardiology* [Internet]. 2008 Mar;51[11]:1112–9.

[38] Shirota K, Huang Y, Kawaguchi O, Yuasa T, Brady PW, Ueda Y, Hunyor SN. Functional recovery of the native heart after cardiomyoplasty in sheep with heart failure: passive and dynamic effects of volume loading. *The Annals of thoracic surgery* [Internet]. 2002 Mar;73[3]:849–54.

[39] Bolotin G, Lorusso R, Schreuder JJ, Nesher N, Kaulbach H, Uretzky G, van der Veen F. Perioperative hemodynamic and geometric changes of the left ventricle during cardiomyoplasty in goats with dilated left ventricle. *Chest* [Internet]. 2002 May;121 [5]:1628–33.

[40] Villarreal D, Freeman RH, Habibullah AA, Simmons JC. Indomethacin attenuates the renal actions of atrial natriuretic factor in dogs with chronic heart failure. *The American journal of the medical sciences* [Internet]. 1997 Aug;314[2]:67–72.

[41] Tessier D, Lajos P, Braunberger E, Pouchelon J-L, Carpentier A, Chachques JC, Chetboul V. Induction of chronic cardiac insufficiency by arteriovenous fistula and doxorubicin administration. *Journal of cardiac surgery* [Internet]. 18[4]:307–11.

[42] Kleaveland JP, Kussmaul WG, Vinciguerra T, Diters R, Carabello BA, Patrick J. Volume overload hypertrophy in a closed-chest model of mitral regurgitation Volume overload hypertrophy model of mitral regurgitation in a closed-chest. 2012;

[43] Zile MR. New Concepts in Diastolic Dysfunction and Diastolic Heart Failure: Part I: Diagnosis, Prognosis, and Measurements of Diastolic Function. *Circulation.* 2002 Mar;105[11]:1387–1393.

[44] Chien SF, Diana JN, Brum JM, Bove a a. A simple technique for producing supra-valvular aortic stenosis in animals. *Cardiovascular research.* 1988 Oct;22[10]:739–45.

[45] Moorjani N, Catarino P, El-Sayed R, Al-Ahmed S, Meyer B, Al-Mohanna F, Westaby S. A pressure overload model to track the molecular biology of heart failure. *European journal of cardio-thoracic surgery : official journal of the European Association for Cardio-thoracic Surgery.* 2003 Dec;24[6]:920–5.

[46] Yarbrough WM, Mukherjee R, Stroud RE, Rivers WT, Oelsen JM, Dixon J a, Eckhouse SR, Ikonomidis JS, Zile MR, Spinale FG. Progressive induction of left ventricular pressure overload in a large animal model elicits myocardial remodeling and a unique matrix signature. *The Journal of thoracic and cardiovascular surgery* [Internet]. 2012 Jan;143[1]:215–23.

[47] Monnet E, Chachques JC. Animal models of heart failure: what is new? *The Annals of thoracic surgery* [Internet]. 2005 Apr;79[4]:1445–53.

[48] Brooks H, Kirk ES, Vokonas PS, Urschel CW, Sonnenblick EH. Performance of the right ventricle under stress: relation to right coronary flow. *The Journal of clinical investigation* [Internet]. 1971 Oct;50[10]:2176–83.

[49] Li B, Yang L, Shen J, Wang C, Jiang Z. The antiproliferative effect of sildenafil on pulmonary artery smooth muscle cells is mediated via upregulation of mitogen-

activated protein kinase phosphatase-1 and degradation of extracellular signal-regulated kinase 1/2 phosphorylation. Anesthesia and analgesia [Internet]. 2007 Oct;105[4]:1034–41, table of contents.

[50] Chen EP, Bittner HB, Tull F, Biswas SS, Davis RD, Van Trigt P. An adult canine model of chronic pulmonary hypertension for cardiopulmonary transplantation. *The Journal of heart and lung transplantation : the official publication of the International Society for Heart Transplantation* [Internet]. 1997 May;16[5]:538–47.

[51] Simon G, Pamnani MB, Dunkel JF, Overbeck HW. Mesenteric hemodynamics in early experimental renal hypertension in dogs. *Circulation Research* [Internet]. 1975 Jun 1;36[6]:791–798.

[52] Morioka S, Simon G. Echocardiographic evidence for early left ventricular hypertrophy in dogs with renal hypertension. *The American journal of cardiology* [Internet]. 1982 Jun;49[8]:1890–5.

[53] Shinbane JS, Wood M a, Jensen DN, Ellenbogen K a, Fitzpatrick a P, Scheinman MM. Tachycardia-induced cardiomyopathy: a review of animal models and clinical studies. *Journal of the American College of Cardiology* [Internet]. 1997 Mar 15;29[4]:709–15.

[54] Frommeyer G, Milberg P, Witte P, Stypmann J, Koopmann M, Lücke M, Osada N, Breithardt G, Fehr M, Eckardt L. A new mechanism preventing proarrhythmia in chronic heart failure: rapid phase-III repolarization explains the low proarrhythmic potential of amiodarone in contrast to sotalol in a model of pacing-induced heart failure. *European journal of heart failure* [Internet]. 2011 Oct;13[10]:1060–9.

[55] Milberg P, Klocke R, Frommeyer G, Quang TH, Dieks K, Stypmann J, Osada N, Kuhlmann M, Fehr M, Milting H, Nikol S, Waltenberger J, Breithardt G, Eckardt L. G-CSF therapy reduces myocardial repolarization reserve in the presence of increased arteriogenesis, angiogenesis and connexin 43 expression in an experimental model of pacing-induced heart failure. *Basic research in cardiology* [Internet]. 2011 Nov;106 [6]:995–1008.

[56] Van Vleet JF, Greenwood LA, Ferrans VJ. Pathologic features of adriamycin toxicosis in young pigs: nonskeletal lesions. *American journal of veterinary research* [Internet]. 1979 Nov;40[11]:1537–52.

[57] Ou L, Li W, Liu Y, Zhang Y, Jie S, Kong D, Steinhoff G, Ma N. Animal models of cardiac disease and stem cell therapy. *The open cardiovascular medicine journal* [Internet]. 2010 Jan;4:231–9.

[58] Toyoda Y, Okada M, Kashem MA. A canine model of dilated cardiomyopathy induced by repetitive intracoronary doxorubicin administration. *The Journal of thoracic and cardiovascular surgery [Internet]*. 1998 Jun;115[6]:1367–73.

[59] Christiansen S, Perez-Bouza A, Schälte G, Hilgers R-D, Autschbach R. Selective left ventricular adriamycin-induced cardiomyopathy in the pig. *The Journal of heart and lung transplantation : the official publication of the International Society for Heart Transplantation* [Internet]. 2008 Jan;27[1]:86–92.

[60] Waters RE, Terjung RL, Peters KG, Annex BH. Preclinical models of human peripheral arterial occlusive disease: implications for investigation of therapeutic agents. J*ournal of applied physiology [Bethesda, Md. : 1985]* [Internet]. 2004 Aug;97[2]:773–80.

[61] LONGLAND CJ. The collateral circulation of the limb; Arris and Gale lecture delivered at the Royal College of Surgeons of England on 4th February, 1953. *Annals of the Royal College of Surgeons of England* [Internet]. 1953 Sep;13[3]:161–76.

[62] Labs JD, Caslowitz PL, Anderson JH, Williams GM. A canine model of controlled thrombotic vascular occlusion. *Investigative radiology* [Internet]. 1989 Jun;24[6]:446–50.

[63] Buschmann IR, Voskuil M, van Royen N, Hoefer IE, Scheffler K, Grundmann S, Hennig J, Schaper W, Bode C, Piek JJ. Invasive and non-invasive evaluation of spontaneous arteriogenesis in a novel porcine model for peripheral arterial obstructive disease. *Atherosclerosis* [Internet]. 2003 Mar;167[1]:33–43.

[64] Powell RJ. Endovascular treatment in the superficial femoral artery: which devices, where? *Seminars in vascular surgery* [Internet]. 2008 Dec;21[4]:180–5.

[65] Houbballah R, Robaldo A, Albadawi H, Titus J, LaMuraglia GM. A novel model of accelerated intimal hyperplasia in the pig iliac artery. I*nternational journal of experimental pathology* [Internet]. 2011 Dec;92[6]:422–7.

[66] Verheye S, Salame MY, Robinson KA, Post MJ, Carrozza JP, Baim DS, Sigwart U, King SB, Chronos NA. Short- and long-term histopathologic evaluation of stenting using a self-expanding nitinol stent in pig carotid and iliac arteries. *Catheterization and cardiovascular interventions : official journal of the Society for Cardiac Angiography & Interventions* [Internet]. 1999 Nov;48[3]:316–23.

[67] Krueger KD, Mitra a K, DelCore MG, Hunter WJ, Agrawal DK. A comparison of stent-induced stenosis in coronary and peripheral arteries. *Journal of clinical pathology* [Internet]. 2006 Jun;59[6]:575–9.

[68] Marmagkiolis K, Hakeem A, Cilingiroglu M, Bailey SR, Ruiz C, Hijazi ZM, Herrmann HC, Zajarias A, Goldberg SL, Feldman T. The society for cardiovascular angiography and interventions structural heart disease early career task force survey results: Endorsed by the society for cardiovascular angiography and interventions. *Catheterization and cardiovascular interventions : official journal of the Society for Cardiac Angiography & Interventions* [Internet]. 2012 Jun 28;:1–11.

[69] Silbiger JJ. Mechanistic insights into ischemic mitral regurgitation: echocardiographic and surgical implications. *Journal of the American Society of Echocardiography : official publication of the American Society of Echocardiography* [Internet]. 2011 Jul;24[7]:707–19.

[70] Trichon BH, Felker GM, Shaw LK, Cabell CH, O'Connor CM. Relation of frequency and severity of mitral regurgitation to survival among patients with left ventricular systolic dysfunction and heart failure. *The American Journal of Cardiology* [Internet]. 2003 Mar;91[5]:538–543.

[71] Yiu SF, Enriquez-Sarano M, Tribouilloy C, Seward JB, Tajik a. J. Determinants of the Degree of Functional Mitral Regurgitation in Patients With Systolic Left Ventricular Dysfunction : *A Quantitative Clinical Study. Circulation* [Internet]. 2000 Sep 19;102[12]:1400–1406.

[72] Kumanohoso T, Otsuji Y, Yoshifuku S, Matsukida K, Koriyama C, Kisanuki A, Minagoe S, Levine R a., Tei C. Mechanism of higher incidence of ischemic mitral regurgitation in patients with inferior myocardial infarction: Quantitative analysis of left ventricular and mitral valve geometry in 103 patients with prior myocardial infarction. *The Journal of Thoracic and Cardiovascular Surgery* [Internet]. 2003 Jan;125[1]:135–143.

[73] Levine R a. Dynamic mitral regurgitation--more than meets the eye. *The New England journal of medicine* [Internet]. 2004 Oct 14;351[16]:1681–4.

[74] Otsuji Y, Handschumacher MD, Liel-Cohen N, Tanabe H, Jiang L, Schwammenthal E, Guerrero JL, Nicholls L a, Vlahakes GJ, Levine R a. Mechanism of ischemic mitral regurgitation with segmental left ventricular dysfunction: three-dimensional echocardiographic studies in models of acute and chronic progressive regurgitation. *Journal of the American College of Cardiology* [Internet]. 2001 Feb;37[2]:641–8.

[75] Tibayan F a, Rodriguez F, Zasio MK, Bailey L, Liang D, Daughters GT, Langer F, Ingels NB, Miller DC. Geometric distortions of the mitral valvular-ventricular complex in chronic ischemic mitral regurgitation. *Circulation* [Internet]. 2003 Sep 9;108 Suppl :II116–21.

[76] Gorman JH, Gorman RC, Jackson BM, Enomoto Y, St. John-Sutton MG, Edmunds LH. Annuloplasty ring selection for chronic ischemic mitral regurgitation: lessons from the ovine model. *The Annals of Thoracic Surgery* [Internet]. 2003 Nov;76[5]:1556–1563.

[77] Joudinaud TM, Kegel CL, Gabster AA, Sanz ML, MacDonald A, Propp D, Callaghan E, Weber PA, Hvass U, Duran CMG. An experimental method for the percutaneous induction of a posterolateral infarct and functional ischemic mitral regurgitation. *The Journal of heart valve disease* [Internet]. 2005 Jul;14[4]:460–6.

[78] Daimon M, Shiota T, Gillinov a M, Hayase M, Ruel M, Cohn WE, Blacker SJ, Liddicoat JR. Percutaneous mitral valve repair for chronic ischemic mitral regurgitation: a real-time three-dimensional echocardiographic study in an ovine model. *Circulation* [Internet]. 2005 May 3;111[17]:2183–9.

[79] Solis J, Levine R a, Johnson B, Guerrero JL, Handschumacher MD, Sullivan S, Lam K, Berlin J, Braithwaite GJC, Muratoglu OK, Vlahakes GJ, Hung J. Polymer injection therapy to reverse remodel the papillary muscles: efficacy in reducing mitral regurgitation in a chronic ischemic model. *Circulation. Cardiovascular interventions* [Internet]. 2010 Oct;3[5]:499–505.

[80] Schmitto JD, Mokashi S a, Lee LS, Laurence R, Schotola H, Coelho-Filho O, Rajab TK, Kwong R, Bolman RM, Quintel M, Cohn LH, Chen FY. A novel, innovative ovine model of chronic ischemic cardiomyopathy induced by multiple coronary ligations. *Artificial organs* [Internet]. 2010 Nov;34[11]:918–22.

[81] Timek TA, Dagum P, Lai DT, Liang D, Daughters GT, Ingels NB, Miller DC. Pathogenesis of mitral regurgitation in tachycardia-induced cardiomyopathy. *Circulation* [Internet]. 2001 Sep 18;104[12 Suppl 1]:I47–53.

[82] Byrne MJ, Raman JS, Alferness CA, Esler MD, Kaye DM, Power JM. An ovine model of tachycardia-induced degenerative dilated cardiomyopathy and heart failure with prolonged onset. *Journal of cardiac failure* [Internet]. 2002 Apr;8[2]:108–15.

[83] Kaye DM, Byrne M, Alferness C, Power J. Feasibility and short-term efficacy of percutaneous mitral annular reduction for the therapy of heart failure-induced mitral regurgitation. *Circulation* [Internet]. 2003 Oct 14;108[15]:1795–7.

[84] Jensen H, Jensen MO, Smerup MH, Ringgaard S, Sørensen TS, Andersen NT, Wierup P, Hasenkam JM, Nielsen SL. Three-dimensional assessment of papillary muscle displacement in a porcine model of ischemic mitral regurgitation. *The Journal of thoracic and cardiovascular surgery* [Internet]. 2010 Dec;140[6]:1312–8.

In: Animal Models in Cancer Research ...
Editor: Sean A. Murray
ISBN: 978-1-62417-587-9

Chapter III

Canine Breast Cancer and Lymphoma as Models in Cancer Research

Farruk Mohammad Lutful Kabir,[1,2] Ann Marie O'Neill,[3] Bruce F. Smith[1,2,4] and Richard Curtis Bird[1,2,*]

[1]Department of Pathobiology, College of Veterinary Medicine, Auburn University, Auburn, Alabama, US

[2]AURIC - Auburn University Research Initiative in Cancer, College of Veterinary Medicine, Auburn University, Auburn, Alabama, US

[3]Department of Nutrition, Dietetics, and Hospitality Management, College of Human Sciences, Auburn University, Auburn, Alabama, US

[4]Scott-Ritchey Research Center, College of Veterinary Medicine, Auburn University, Auburn, Alabama, US

Abstract

While tumors in companion animals (dogs and cats) draw attention in the realm of pet care, they also offer unique opportunities to develop valid models in which to study human cancers and translational cancer therapeutics. Spontaneous tumors in dogs are appropriate intermediate model systems for a number of reasons. Dogs represent an outbred population that has a shared environment with humans. Canine cancers often demonstrate similar histopathologic and biologic behavior to tumors occurring in humans, and the size of the model allows for extrapolation to humans. Canine mammary carcinoma and lymphoma are two excellent examples of tumors that have potential relevance to human cancer biology. Canine malignant mammary tumors are very common in middle aged, sexually intact female dogs and have a metastatic pattern similar to that in women. Moreover, mammary carcinomas in female dogs provide a high level of similarity in genetics, pathology and environmental exposure when compared to human

[*] Telephone: 334-844-2707, Fax: 334-844-2652, E-mail: birdric@auburn.edu.

breast cancer. Like humans, expression of canine cell proliferation and cell cycle regulatory genes are frequently altered in breast cancer. Lymphoma is a highly aggressive disease of dogs and is one of the most common tumors seen in the domestic dog. Middle-to-old age dogs are more often affected, with certain breeds showing increased incidence. The most common clinical presentation in dogs is similar to non-Hodgkin's lymphoma (NHL) in humans and as such has been proposed as a model for human disease. This canine model is further supported by the presence of evolutionarily conserved cytogenetic changes. Adding to the power of both canine breast cancer and lymphoma is the high similarity between dog and human genomes, allowing comparative genomics approaches to understanding these tumors and potential response to therapy.

1. Introduction

Cancer is one of the leading causes of death in both humans and companion animals such as dogs and cats. It is a complex biologic process especially in terms of greater heterogeneity and genetic deregulation the natural consequences of which cause deadly features of this disease including acquiring resistance to therapy, recurrent invasion and metastasis. Comprehensive experimental model systems are highly valued for the study of human cancers. A number of important advancements in oncology have been made possible by employing animal models that represent many aspects of the complexity of human cancers, allowing understanding of molecular mechanisms of cancer and eventually leading to the development of new cancer therapeutics.

Animal models play crucial roles in the design of laboratory experiments in biomedical research. These models are especially important for providing evidence from experimental evaluation, establishing preclinical safety and efficacy necessary for progressing to human clinical trials. Although *in vivo* rodent models such as xenografts and transgenics have been widely used in human cancer research, they have intrinsic limitations in terms of management, specific biological characteristics, pathology, genetics and induced laboratory conditions [1]. Most murine models must be induced in the laboratory to mimic cellular and molecular features of human cancers. These models have been demonstrated to fail in recapitulating essential features of human cancers such as significant heterogeneity in tumor cells, tumor microenvironment, regulation of the immune system, genetic manipulation and intricate molecular mechanisms involving a vast network of cancer related genes [2,3]. In addition to induced genetic modification and lack of spontaneous oncogenic features in transgenic mice, intrinsic evolutionary distance between mice and humans can pose challenges when comparing murine models to study human cancers. The hunt for appropriate animal models in cancer research has steered scientists to consider companion animals (pet dogs and cats) with spontaneously occurring neoplasms as valuable and still largely under-utilized resources.

1.1. Dogs as Appropriate Animal Models of Human Cancers

In the field of human cancer research, there is an increased propensity to examine the value of new experimental models in terms of similarities with human malignancies and therefore to select more appropriate animal models that better define the complex biology of cancers in human patients. In this regard, companion animals display many desired characteristics that bridge between *in vivo* small animal model and human studies. Among pet animals, domesticated dogs (*Canis lupus familiaris*) are considered excellent preclinical models of cancers and other complex human diseases for many reasons, including their easy accessibility, common and prominent status in diverse cultures [4]. Most of these pet dogs experience a shared environment with their owners (either for living or environmental risk factors) [5,6] which is an important feature exploited by scientists investigating cancer etiologies. Additionally, dogs represent a more outbred population than inbred laboratory animals providing a genetic diversity similar to that seen in humans [7].

Because of the high quality of the entire dog genome sequence (~2.5 billion base pairs similar in size to the human genome) and the identification of nearly all of its genes as clear orthologs of known human genes, the dog has emerged as an exceptional model for the study of human cancers [7]. For many gene families associated with cancer, the similarities between dog and human have been found to be significantly closer than the relationship between mouse and human [8]. Importantly, there are strong similarities in clinical and molecular features between human and canine cancers. Like humans, dogs spontaneously develop cancers with a clinical presentation, histologic morphology, tumor genetics, molecular targets, biologic behavior, disease progression and response to conventional therapies that is highly comparable [9-11]. Moreover, cancers naturally develop in dog in the context of an intact immune system where tumor, host and tumor microenvironment are syngeneic [10]. Many histological types of cancer are also associated with similar genetic alterations in humans and dogs. There are significant overlapping regions of the human and canine genomes that are frequently disrupted and correlated with cancer progression suggesting a strong and similar genetic predisposition in both species [12].

Canine tumors with potential relevance for human cancer biology include osteosarcoma, mammary carcinoma, lymphoma, oral melanoma, lung carcinoma, and soft tissue sarcomas [11]. Canine mammary carcinoma and lymphoma are highly prevalent and life-threatening cancers in all dogs [13-15]. These canine cancers provide a high level of similarity in cytogenetics, pathology and environmental exposure when compared to their human counterparts [16-18].

2. Canine Mammary Tumor Model

Mammary cancers are the most common tumors in sexually intact middle-aged female dogs. Approximately 50% of all these neoplasms are diagnosed as malignant [13,14,19]. Breast tumors represent the second most frequent neoplasms in dogs and humans after skin and lung cancers, respectively, although the incidence of mammary cancer in female dogs tends to be higher than the incidence in women in certain geographical area [20-22]. A large number of studies have demonstrated that canine mammary tumors (CMT) have many similarities with breast cancer in humans supporting the use of dogs as valuable comparative and predictive intermediate models for human breast cancer. Most of the cancer-associated genetic alterations critical to mammary tumor development and metastasis are also similar in both species. Gene expression analysis has revealed a significant overlap in canine and human genes that are deregulated or defective in mammary tumors compared with normal mammary tissue. Cell proliferation in normal epithelium is tightly controlled by several regulators of the cell cycle check points [23]. Uncontrolled cellular proliferation is the hallmark of neoplastic transformation of mammary tissue. In this regard, CMT cells have defective expression of cell cycle regulatory genes (often called tumor suppressors) and abnormal expression of oncogenes that promote cellular transformation and tumor development. Like humans, expression of canine cell proliferation and cell cycle regulatory genes are frequently altered in CMTs [13,17,24]. Genome wide comparative analysis has also demonstrated that genes involved in increased proliferative activity in mammary tumors in both humans and dogs are upregulated whereas genes related to cell development, cell communication and cell matrix adhesion are downregulated [25]. A comparative analysis of gene expression and defects in both species therefore strongly support canine mammary tumors as valuable intermediate models for human breast cancer.

Table 1. Differential expression of INK4 genes in CMT cell lines

	p16/INK4A	p14ARF	p15/INK4B	p18/INK4C	p19/INK4D
CMT9	-	+	+	++	++
CMT12	-	-	-	++	++
CMT27	-	-	-	++	++
CMT28	+*	+	+	++	++
CMT47	-	-	+	++	++
CMT119	-	-	-	++	++
NCF (normal canine fibroblast)	+	+	+	+	+

(-) No expression; (+) normal expression; (++) overexpression.
* Novel deletion in exon 1α.

2.1. Expression Defects of Cell Cycle Regulators in the CMT Model

Cell cycle progression is a highly regulated process and governed by a number of proteins called cyclin/cyclin-dependent kinases (CDKs) whose activities are controlled by cyclin-dependent kinase inhibitors (CKIs) [26,27]. Based on their sequence similarity and specific roles in cell cycle regulation, CKIs are divided into two distinct families: the INK4 family (p16/INK4A, p14ARF, p15/INK4B, p18/INK4C and p19/INK4D) and the CIP/KIP family (p21/CIP1, p27/KIP1 and p57/KIP2) [28,29]. All of the CKIs are proven tumor suppressor genes, or suspected of having this potential, since mutations in these genes promote a malignant phenotype [30,31]. These two CKI families have distinct cell cycle regulatory as well as tumor suppressive functions. Members of the INK4 family CKIs inhibit CDK4 and CDK6 association with cyclin D, preventing Rb phosphorylation and thereby inactivating the E2F transcription factor required for expression of numerous genes involved in the G1 to S phase transition [32]. On the other hand, CIP/KIPs inhibit a number of cyclin-CDK complexes such as cyclin E-CDK2, cyclin D-CDK4 and cyclin A-CDK2 involved in G1 to S phase transition [33-36]. Recent studies have reported that both the INK4 and CIP/KIP families are differentially expressed in a panel of different canine mammary tumor cell lines. Among INK4 CKIs, p16, p14ARF and p15 are most frequently found to be defective in CMT cell lines (Table 1) [37,24], while expression of p21 and p27 of the CIP/KIP family and also the tumor suppressor p53 which acts as transcriptional activator of p21, are deregulated (either overexpressed or not expressed) in CMT cell lines [37,17,38].

p53 is one of the best characterized tumor suppressors and a master regulator of cell cycle, proliferation, DNA repair and autophagy and is activated in response to DNA damage or oxidative stress and leads to irreversible cell cycle arrest [39]. Recent studies reported that p53-dependent cellular mechanisms prevent malignant transformation of cells rendering human mammary epithelium resistant to tumorigenesis [40,41]. Importantly, in mammary carcinomas, a similar altered expression profile of p53 was identified in both humans and dogs, suggesting equivalent roles in carcinogenesis and potential use as a prognostic marker [42,43]. p53-induced cell cycle arrest is mediated by a transcriptional increase of the cyclin dependent kinase inhibitor p21 which can be overexpressed in some canine mammary carcinomas when compared to other metastases [44] although there is some question as to whether overexpression is necessary [37,17]. Increased expression of p21 in metastatic mammary tumors is thought to be a p53-induced attempt to inhibit cell cycle progression that fails in at least some tumors [45].

Deregulation of p16/INK4A/ARF/INK4B Locus in CMTs

The regions of the human chromosome 9p21 and dog chromosome 11 that harbor the INK4A/ARF/INK4B locus have been reported to be frequently disrupted in both human and canine cancers [24,46,47]. Loss of this locus is one of the most recurrent cytogenetic events in a wide spectrum of human cancers [48]. The INK4A/ARF/INK4B locus encodes three related genes - p16/INK4A, p14ARF and p15/INK4B that play widespread and independent roles in tumor suppression [48,49]. Whereas p15/INK4B has its own reading frame and is physically distinct, p16/INK4A and p14ARF share a common second and third exon but each has a different and unique first exon (exon 1α and 1β, respectively). The two transcripts (p16/INK4A and p14ARF) resulting from alternative splicing of the gene are then translated from alternative reading frames making two different proteins with distinct functions [48,50,51]. Although they have a large overlapping nucleotide sequence, they function in different anti-proliferative pathways. p16 inhibits G1/S phase transition by inhibiting CDK4/6-cyclin D1 complexes [52] while p14ARF stabilizes p53 protein disrupting interactions with the E3 ubiquitin ligase mdm2[53].

Both p16 and p14ARF are important candidates for the study of novel cancer mechanisms. The potent tumor suppressor activity of the INK4A/AFR/INK4B locus has been confirmed by knockout studies showing that mice deficient for p16 and p14ARF (or p19ARF for in mice) are more prone to spontaneous cancers compared to wild type littermates [54]. A great number of tumors have been examined to determine the most important member among the products of the INK4A/AFR/INK4B locus in the absence of mutation of the others. Such studies evaluated p16/INK4A as the most potent tumor suppressor member of the locus [54], defects in which are strongly associated with tumor susceptibility [55] and its lesions are second in frequency only to p53 for human malignancies [56]. Studies of numerous human cancers have reported specific somatic loss of p16 through point mutation or small deletions [57] and also more frequent germline mutations in p16 have been detected compared to p14ARF and p15 [58]. A large number of human cancers have also been analyzed and determined to have epigenetic mutations or promoter hypermethylation in the p16 gene [59]. Additionally, experimental evidence has shown that p16 can act as a potent growth suppressor and specific inhibitor of the G1/S phase transition. Introduction of full length human p16 cDNA caused marked growth suppression through accumulation of cells in G1 phase in p16 knockout human glioma [60], lung cancer [61], esophageal cancer cells [62] as well as in human and canine breast cancer cells [63,37]. All this evidence unquestionably points to p16 as an important tumor suppressor in human and canine cancers.

The unusual genomic rearrangement of the INK4A/ARF/INK4B locus is certainly a critical area of research where we need to improve our understanding for deciphering the molecular mechanism encoded in this gene locus. Unlike humans, canine p16 and p14ARF derived from the INK4 locus have not been fully elucidated. Lack of full-length mRNA sequence or expressed sequence tags and presence of highly GC-rich sequences have made it difficult to clone or sequence, causing a gap in the CanFam 2.0 canine genome assembly [7]. Recent studies have reported differential and defective expression patterns for p16 in several spontaneous canine mammary tumor cell lines [37,24]. The same expression profile was also evaluated in primary mammary cells isolated from several canine tumor biopsy samples suggesting that the gene expression defects were not an artifact of *in vitro* cell culture. Importantly, the complete coding region of p16 has been sequenced, analyzed and compared with the same locus in normal canine fibroblasts (NCF) [24]. The canine p16 sequence was then aligned with human and other mammalian p16 sequences showing that they are highly conserved across the mammals. Most strikingly, the p16 sequence from a CMT cell line was discovered to harbor a novel frameshift mutation resulting from a small 17 bp deletion in exon 1α of p16. Interestingly, this mapping of the mutation can directly be compared to human p16 where most recurrent deletions also center on exon 1α and exon 2 of INK4A gene [48]. Moreover, the frameshift mutation in p16 in the CMT model, altered the reading frame and shifting it to that of p14ARF (from the exon 1 and 2 boundary) resulting in a putatively truncated and chimeric protein [24]. The frameshift mutation has been predicted to disrupt the protein native folding and functional integrity supporting previous experimental evidence that the same CMT model does not express detectable p16 protein [64].

2.2. Genome-Wide Comparative Analysis of the Role of Critical Genes Involved in Human and Canine Mammary Tumors

Genome-wide comparative analysis of gene expression revealed that a significant number of genes that are known to be differentially expressed in human breast cancer are also deregulated in the canine mammary tumor model. Changes in gene expression levels from independent human and dog microarray studies have been compared and mapped for orthologous gene sets represented across both microarray platforms. This high-throughput analysis showed that clustering of altered gene expression largely depends on the metastatic stages and origin of tumor samples implying a close overall transcriptional similarity of signature genes between human and canine mammary tumors [25].A pathway focused analysis of these genes uncovered a large degree of similarity in the regulation of several cancer related pathways, such as the phosphatidylinositol 3 kinase (PI3K)/AKT pathway, the K-RAS, phosphatase and tensin homolog (PTEN), the Wnt-β, catenin and the mitogen activated protein kinase (MAPK) pathways.

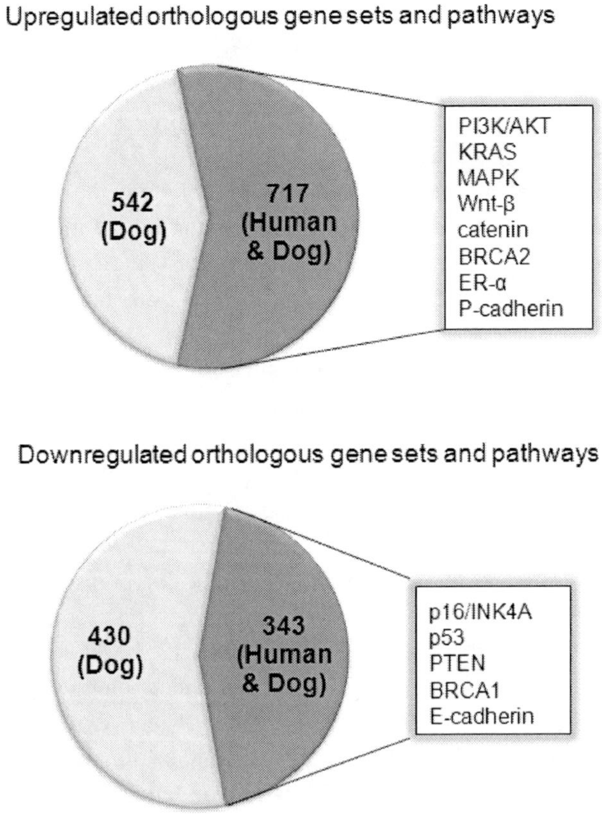

Figure 1. Up/down-regulated orthologous gene sets and signaling pathways in human and canine mammary tumors. In the upper panel, prominent oncogenic pathways and related genes (shown in rectangular box on right) belong to 717 upregulated orthologous genes in humans and dogs out of 1259 genes identified in breast cancer. In the lower panel, representative tumor suppressive pathways and related genes (shown in lower rectangular box on right) are included in 343 downregulated orthologs out of 773 genes. This analysis of abnormally regulated cancer associated genes or pathways is based on a number of recent studies in the field of canine breast cancer [24,25,42,44,65-69].

Comparative analysis of deregulated gene sets or cancer signaling pathways showed that a significant proportion of orthologous genes are comparably up- and downregulated in both human and dog breast tumors. As many as 717 out of 1259 orthologous genes are upregulated and 343 out of 773 orthologous genes are downregulated in both species (Figure 1) [25,65].

The PI3K/AKT pathway plays a critical role in the regulation of cellular transformation, growth, proliferation, and survival and its aberrant activation has been implicated in the development and progression of a number of cancers [66,67]. Upregulation of the PI3K/AKT pathway in CMT is thought to be stimulated by activation of several genes in this pathway. The loss of PTEN has been attributed as a signature in both human and canine mammary tumors and is reported to be a strong activator of the PI3K/AKT pathway [66,25]. PTEN is considered to be a gatekeeper tumor suppressor gene with prognostic relevance for CMT as evidence has shown an association between loss of PTEN expression and significantly shorter survival times for dogs with malignant mammary tumors [68,45]. PTEN is involved in multiple cellular mechanisms, including important roles in inhibition of proliferation, induction of apoptosis and cell adhesion that may lead to cellular defense against neoplastic transformation [45]. Another oncogenic signaling pathway upstream of PI3K/AKT, called K-

RAS is also upregulated in canine and human breast cancers [69,25]. Oncogenic K-RAS is an activated GTP-bound form that is constitutively activated by somatic mutation in many cancers including breast cancer [69,67]. The mitogen activated protein kinase (MAPK) signaling pathway also regulates a variety of cellular processes such as gene expression, mitosis, differentiation, cell survival and apoptosis [70]. The MAPKpathway involves a complex network of interactions between proteins, including the activation of the K-RAS protein and the inactivation of components of the cellular apoptotic machinery. Genes in this signaling pathway that act as tumor suppressors involved in regulation of cellular proliferation and inducing apoptosis, are all downregulated in both human and canine mammary tumors [70,25].

The Wnt-β catenin pathway is a complex network of proteins widely known for their crucial role in embryonic development in all animal species. Wnt, part of a highly controlled signaling pathway in normal developmental processes, also plays an important role in the regulation of cellular proliferation [71]. However, the Wnt pathway can also play a central role in cancer because of the fact that many genes in this developmental pathway can act as oncogenes or tumor suppressors [72].

Comparative gene expression analysis of human and dog breast tumors demonstrated that many of the Wnt signaling components that act as tumor suppressors are downregulated and thereby globally activate pathways to breast cancer [25]. Another study reported that epigenetic silencing of Wnt-antagonist genes, by frequent methylation, triggers the same pathway in human breast cancer [73]. Similar altered gene expression profiles and Wnt pathway activation has been delineated in canine mammary tumors [74]. Taken together, this close and promising resemblance in the regulation of target genes and critical molecular signaling pathways involved in mammary tumors in both species supports the use of spontaneous canine mammary tumors as a valuable and predictive intermediate model for human breast cancer.

2.3. Expression of miRNAs in Human Breast Cancer and the CMT Model

MicroRNAs (miRNAs) are evolutionarily conserved, endogenous small noncoding RNA molecules (~22 nucleotides) that post-transcriptionally suppress gene expression in a sequence specific manner [75]. Expression of these small RNAs is tightly regulated during development and in normal tissues and is frequently altered in cancer [76].

More than 50% of miRNA genes are located in cancer associated genomic regions or fragile sites that are also preferential sites for translocation, deletion, amplification, and integration of exogenous genome fragments suggesting that miRNAs play an important role in the pathogenesis of many human cancers [77]. Since miRNAs are encoded by highly conserved naturally occurring genes across mammalian species, evaluation of their expression profiles in an animal model comparable to human might expedite their development of future therapeutic reagents.

miRNAs are often regarded as 'oncomirs' (either as tumor suppressors or oncogenes) since their aberrant expression has been associated with the development of different pathologies, including cancer. A large number of miRNAs have been identified as deregulated in human breast cancer compared to normal breast tissue. Several miRNAs are downregulated that are thought to act as tumor suppressors including miR-10b, miR-125b and miR-145.

While oncogenic miRNAs that are significantly upregulated in breast cancer include miR-21 and miR-155 [78]. It can be expected that targets of downregulated miRNAs are likely oncogenes or genes that switch on oncogenic functions. On the other hand, upregulated miRNAs might target tumor suppressors or genes involved in restraining proliferation and promoting apoptosis. Evidence has shown that miR-21 simultaneously regulates the expression of many anti-metastatic genes.

For example, in human breast cancer, miR-21 targets PTEN [79] thereby activating the PI3K/ATK signaling pathway, tropomyosin 1 (TPM1) [80], programmed cell death-4 (PDCD4) [81,82], Bcl2 [83] and TGF-β [78]. Interestingly, all of these miR-21 targets have been reported to be deregulated in canine mammary tumors. In this regard, expression of ten miRNAs associated with human breast cancers were investigated in canine malignant mammary tumors. Almost all of the miRNAs followed the same expression pattern observed in human breast cancers when compared to normal canine mammary tissue. This investigation revealed that miR-21 and miR-29b were significantly upregulated and miR-15b, miR-16 were significantly downregulated in breast cancers in both species [84].

3. Canine Lymphoma Model

Neoplasms originating from the cells of the lymphopoietic system encompass a diverse group of cancers that are collectively known as lymphomas and account for around 5% of all human cancers in the United States (Cancer trends progress reports 2006). Lymphoma alone represents over 50% of all neoplasms that affect bone marrow, blood cells, lymph nodes and other parts of the lymphatic system [85]. Lymphoma diagnosis is based on the World Health Organization (WHO) classification and subdivided into Hodgkin and non-Hodgkin lymphomas (NHL). It is estimated that there will be over 70,000 new cases of NHL in the US in 2012 (see http://cancer.gov /cancertopics/types/non-hodgkin). The majority of human patients are over 60 years of age, with more men than women affected. Since the 1970's, the incidence of the disease has been rising although the etiology is not fully understood [86], thus an alternative model is required to elucidate the causes and biology of lymphoma.

Canine NHL is a naturally occurring, spontaneous disease of dogs that is similar to human NHL in terms of pathology and course of disease. This is the most common lymphoma of dogs, accounting for over 80% of canine hematopoietic neoplasms. The disease affects mainly middle to old age dogs, with certain breeds showing an increased incidence although all breeds and ages are affected [87].

The most prevalent NHL type is the same in humans and dogs characterizing diffuse large B cells. The incidence of canine lymphoma is approximately five times that of the human disease [88,89] and this may be due, in part, to the prevalence of the disease in certain dog breeds and the variation in the prevalence of either B or T cell disease in different breeds [90,91]. While this suggests a link between lymphoma and genetic factors, the breed prevalence also provides an opportunity to identify genetic factors that may be important in tumorigenesis and progression in a model that has the potential to avoid the heterogeneity that may confound human studies [92].

NHL refers to a heterogeneous group of diseases that can arise from B, T or NK cells at different stages of maturation of the cells of origin [93]. The majority of human NHLs (85-

90%) are of B lymphocyte origin. In order to classify lymphomas, a number of systems have been devised over the years however recently the revised WHO system has been developed and diagnosis incorporates recent clinical and laboratory finding into the description. The feasibility of using this system in canine lymphoma diagnosis has been assessed and the same criteria that are used to define disease in humans can be used, with excellent reproducibility of results, to define the disease in the dog [94].

The most common subtype of NHL is diffuse large B cell lymphoma (DLBCL) which describes a group of disorders with a number of subtypes [86]. Similar to the human disease, canine NHL is initially responsive to chemotherapy however relapse and chemoresistance is common. Over-expression of a number of proteins that are implicated in drug resistance including the transport protein P-glycoprotein (P-gp) has been described in the human disease [95]. Expression of P-gp has been reported in a number of studies in cases of relapsed and chemoresistant canine lymphomas [96-99].

Genomic imbalance has been well documented in human lymphoma and a number of similar chromosomal aberrations have been identified in the canine disease. In humans, translocation of the MYC oncogene from HSA8q4 to 14q32 results in fusion with the immunoglobulin enhancer and transcriptional dysregulation [100,16].

Aberrations identified in the canine disease appear to be confined to chromosomes 13 and 31 and include the gain of CFA 13 and the gain of CFA 31. These aneuploidies are analogous to the gain of HSA21 and partial gain of HSA4 in human NHL, resulting in the presence of a MYC-IGH (Immunoglobin heavy chain) like translocation [101-103,16].

The role of miRNAs and their involvement in canine lymphoma has also been the subject of recent studies. The role of miRNAs in post-transcriptional regulation and involvement in the development of tumors has been demonstrated in a number of studies of the human disease [104]. Increased expression of miR-19a+b and miR-17-5p, which upregulate oncogenes, and decreased expression of miR-203, miR-218 and miR-181a that have known tumor suppression functions, has been demonstrated in a number of canine lymphoid cell lines and lymphomas, [105,106]. Nevertheless, this data suggests that this is an area that requires further research as there is clearly potential for both oncogenic and tumor suppressor potential among those few miRNAs identified to date.

Conclusion

The strong similarities in genome sequence, along with highly similar characteristics for several spontaneous tumor types, have raised great promise for further comparative research between humans and dogs. Among several shared tumor types these two species both suffer from breast cancer and lymphoma and recent developments have promoted these canine tumors as attractive intermediate animal models in human cancer research. Comparing mammary carcinomas in female dogs with breast cancer in women has greatly improved our understanding of the molecular mechanisms, relevant risk factors and genetic profiles of this type of cancer. Like mammary tumors, lymphomas in dogs also display clinical features, genomic susceptibility or chromosomal dysregulation and responses to chemotherapy that are similar to humans. Although there is great potential in canine cancer models, a large number of cancer associated genes have not yet been well studied in these species. There has also been an increased need for dog specific genome-wide arrays to study disease phenotypes. These high resolution genome-wide association (GWAS) studies have been widely used to identify major cancer susceptibility genes and can contribute to early diagnosis and also assist in the development of novel therapeutics. In the post-GWAS era massively parallel sequencing, a next generation sequencing technology, has demonstrated a higher level of complexity to the human genome with respect to new genetic variations including single nucleotide polymorphisms (SNPs), small insertions and deletions (indels) and copy number variation [107]. This technique has already been applied in human breast cancer replacing the classical candidate gene approaches to identify novel breast cancer susceptibility genes [108]. Although geneticists have started using this sequencing technology for the genome analysis of the domestic dog [109], it is yet to be explored in canine cancer models. By applying these high-throughput approaches to the dog genome to mine novel candidate genes, including genes that may potentiate neoplasia but not directly cause it as well as associated biomarkers, elucidation of the intricate molecular mechanisms in canine mammary tumor and lymphoma models should be advanced. Such advances and the development of canine therapeutic strategies have enormous potential in the development of future therapeutics for similar human cancers.

References

[1] De Vico G, Maiolino P, Restucci B, Passantino A (2005). Spontaneous tumours of pet dog as models for human cancers: searching for adequate guidelines. *Riv. Biol.* 98 (2) 279-296.

[2] Hansen K, Khanna C (2004). Spontaneous and genetically engineered animal models; use in preclinical cancer drug development. *Eur. J. Cancer,* 40 (6) 858-880.

[3] Nandi S, Guzman RC, Yang J (1995). Hormones and mammary carcinogenesis in mice, rats, and humans: a unifying hypothesis. *Proc. Natl. Acad Sci. U S A* 92 (9) 3650-3657.

[4] Rowell JL, McCarthy DO, Alvarez CE (2011). Dog models of naturally occurring cancer. *Trends Mol. Med.* 17 (7) 380-388.

[5] Smith BF, Bird RC (2010). Hematologic Neoplasia - Gene Therapy. In: Weiss DJ, Wardrop KJ (eds) Schalm's Veterinary Hematology, (550-557), Iowa, Wiley-Blackwell.

[6] American Veterinary Medical Association (2008). US pet ownership and demographics sourcebook 2007, Schaumburg, Illinois, American Veterinary Medical Association.

[7] Lindblad-Toh K, Wade CM, Mikkelsen TS, Karlsson EK, Jaffe DB, Kamal M, Clamp M et al. (2005). Genome sequence, comparative analysis and haplotype structure of the domestic dog. *Nature* 438 (7069) 803-819.

[8] Hoffman MM, Birney E (2007). Estimating the neutral rate of nucleotide substitution using introns. *Mol. Biol. Evol.* 24 (2) 522-531.

[9] Khanna C, Lindblad-Toh K, Vail D, London C, Bergman P, Barber L, Breen M et al. (2006). The dog as a cancer model. *Nat. Biotechnol.* 24 (9) 1065-1066.

[10] Paoloni M, Khanna C (2008). Translation of new cancer treatments from pet dogs to humans. *Nat. Rev. Cancer,*8 (2) 147-156.

[11] Vail DM, MacEwen EG (2000). Spontaneously occurring tumors of companion animals as models for human cancer. *Cancer Invest.* 18 (8) 781-792.

[12] Tang J, Le S, Sun L, Yan X, Zhang M, Macleod J, Leroy B et al. (2010). Copy number abnormalities in sporadic canine colorectal cancers. *Genome Res.* 20 (3) 341-350.

[13] Ahern TE, Bird RC, Bird AE, Wolfe LG (1996). Expression of the oncogene c-erbB-2 in canine mammary cancers and tumor-derived cell lines. *Am. J. Vet. Res.* 57 (5) 693-696.

[14] Rutteman GR, Withrow SJ, MacEwen EG (2001). Tumors of the mammary gland. In: Withrow SJ, MacEwen EG (eds) *Small Animal Clinical Oncology*, (455-477), Philadelphia, WB Saunders.

[15] Shearin AL, Ostrander EA (2010). Leading the way: canine models of genomics and disease. *Dis. Model Mech.* 3 (1-2) 27-34.

[16] Breen M, Modiano JF (2008). Evolutionarily conserved cytogenetic changes in hematological malignancies of dogs and humans--man and his best friend share more than companionship. *Chromosome Res.* 16 (1) 145-154.

[17] DeInnocentes P, Li LX, Sanchez RL, Bird RC (2006). Expression and sequence of canine SIRT2 and p53 genes in canine mammary tumour cells - effects on downstream targets Wip1 and p21/Cip1. *Vet. Comp. Oncol.* 4 (3) 161-177.

[18] Migone F, Deinnocentes P, Smith BF, Bird RC (2006). Alterations in CDK1 expression and nuclear/nucleolar localization following induction in a spontaneous canine mammary cancer model. *J. Cell Biochem.* 98 (3) 504-518.

[19] Withrow SJ, MacEwen EG (1996). Small animal clinical oncology, Philadelphia, WB Saunders.

[20] Jemal A, Siegel R, Ward E, Murray T, Xu J, Thun MJ (2007). Cancer statistics, 2007. *CA Cancer J. Clin.* 57 (1) 43-66.

[21] Owen LN (1979). A comparative study of canine and human breast cancer. *Invest. Cell Pathol.* 2 (4) 257-275.

[22] Sorenmo K (2003). Canine mammary gland tumors. *Vet. Clin. North Am. Small Anim. Pract.* 33 (3) 573-596.

[23] Sarli G, Preziosi R, Benazzi C, Castellani G, Marcato PS (2002). Prognostic value of histologic stage and proliferative activity in canine malignant mammary tumors. *J. Vet. Diagn. Invest.*14 (1) 25-34.

[24] Lutful Kabir FM, Agarwal P, Deinnocentes P, Zaman J, Bird AC, Bird RC (2012). Novel frameshift mutation in the p16/INK4A tumor suppressor gene in canine breast cancer alters expression from the p16/INK4A/p14ARF locus. *J. Cell Biochem.*114 (1) 56-66.

[25] Uva P, Aurisicchio L, Watters J, Loboda A, Kulkarni A, Castle J, Palombo F et al. (2009). Comparative expression pathway analysis of human and canine mammary tumors. *BMC Genomics* 10135.

[26] Morgan DO (1997). Cyclin-dependent kinases: engines, clocks, and microprocessors. *Annu. Rev. Cell Dev. Biol.* 13261-291.

[27] Pines J, Hunter T (1991). Cyclin-dependent kinases: a new cell cycle motif? *Trends Cell Biol.* 1 (5) 117-121.

[28] Sherr CJ, Roberts JM (1999). CDK inhibitors: positive and negative regulators of G1-phase progression. *Genes Dev.* 13 (12) 1501-1512.

[29] Vidal A, Koff A (2000). Cell-cycle inhibitors: three families united by a common cause. *Gene,* 247 (1-2) 1-15.

[30] Kinzler KW, Vogelstein B (1997). Cancer-susceptibility genes. Gatekeepers and caretakers. *Nature,* 386 (6627) 761, 763.

[31] Tripathy D, Benz CC (1992). Activated oncogenes and putative tumor suppressor genes involved in human breast cancers. *Cancer Treat Res*. 6315-60.

[32] Weinberg RA (1995). The retinoblastoma protein and cell cycle control. *Cell,* 81 (3) 323-330.

[33] Harper JW, Adami GR, Wei N, Keyomarsi K, Elledge SJ (1993). The p21 Cdk-interacting protein Cip1 is a potent inhibitor of G1 cyclin-dependent kinases. *Cell,* 75 (4) 805-816.

[34] Lee MH, Reynisdottir I, Massague J (1995). Cloning of p57KIP2, a cyclin-dependent kinase inhibitor with unique domain structure and tissue distribution. *Genes Dev*. 9 (6) 639-649.

[35] Polyak K, Kato JY, Solomon MJ, Sherr CJ, Massague J, Roberts JM, Koff A (1994). p27Kip1, a cyclin-Cdk inhibitor, links transforming growth factor-beta and contact inhibition to cell cycle arrest. *Genes Dev*.8 (1) 9-22.

[36] Toyoshima H, Hunter T (1994). p27, a novel inhibitor of G1 cyclin-Cdk protein kinase activity, is related to p21. Cell 78 (1) 67-74.

[37] DeInnocentes P, Agarwal P, Bird RC (2009). Phenotype-rescue of cyclin-dependent kinase inhibitor p16/INK4A defects in a spontaneous canine cell model of breast cancer. *J. Cell Biochem.* 106 (3) 491-505.

[38] Levine AJ (1997). p53, the cellular gatekeeper for growth and division. *Cell,* 88 (3) 323-331.

[39] Vousden KH, Prives C (2009). Blinded by the Light: The Growing Complexity of p53. *Cell,* 137 (3) 413-431.

[40] Jerry DJ, Dunphy KA, Hagen MJ (2010). Estrogens, regulation of p53 and breast cancer risk: a balancing act. *Cell Mol. Life Sci.* 67 (7) 1017-1023

[41] Millau JF, Bastien N, Drouin R (2009). P53 transcriptional activities: a general overview and some thoughts. *Mutat. Res.* 681 (2-3) 118-133.

[42] Haga S, Nakayama M, Tatsumi K, Maeda M, Imai S, Umesako S, Yamamoto H et al. (2001). Overexpression of the p53 gene product in canine mammary tumors. *Oncol. Rep.* 8 (6) 1215-1219.

[43] Rungsipipat A, Tateyama S, Yamaguchi R, Uchida K, Miyoshi N, Hayashi T (1999). Immunohistochemical analysis of c-yes and c-erbB-2 oncogene products and p53 tumor suppressor protein in canine mammary tumors. *J. Vet. Med. Sci.*61 (1) 27-32.

[44] Klopfleisch R, Gruber AD (2009). Differential expression of cell cycle regulators p21, p27 and p53 in metastasizing canine mammary adenocarcinomas versus normal mammary glands. *Res. Vet. Sci.* 87 (1) 91-96.

[45] Klopfleisch R, von Euler H, Sarli G, Pinho SS, Gartner F, Gruber AD (2011). Molecular carcinogenesis of canine mammary tumors: news from an old disease. *Vet. Pathol.* 48 (1) 98-116.

[46] Ruas M, Peters G (1998). The p16INK4a/CDKN2A tumor suppressor and its relatives. *Biochim. Biophys. Acta,* 1378 (2) F115-177.

[47] Sharpless NE (2005). INK4a/ARF: a multifunctional tumor suppressor locus. *Mutat. Res.* 576 (1-2) 22-38.

[48] Kim WY, Sharpless NE (2006). The regulation of INK4/ARF in cancer and aging. *Cell,* 127 (2) 265-275.

[49] Sherr CJ (2000). The Pezcoller lecture: cancer cell cycles revisited. *Cancer Res.* 60 (14) 3689-3695.
[50] Quelle DE, Zindy F, Ashmun RA, Sherr CJ (1995). Alternative reading frames of the INK4a tumor suppressor gene encode two unrelated proteins capable of inducing cell cycle arrest. *Cell,* 83 (6) 993-1000.
[51] Stone S, Jiang P, Dayananth P, Tavtigian SV, Katcher H, Parry D, Peters G et al. (1995). Complex structure and regulation of the P16 (MTS1) locus. *Cancer Res.* 55 (14) 2988-2994.
[52] Russo AA, Tong L, Lee JO, Jeffrey PD, Pavletich NP (1998). Structural basis for inhibition of the cyclin-dependent kinase Cdk6 by the tumour suppressor p16INK4a. *Nature*, 395 (6699) 237-243.
[53] Boehme KA, Blattner C (2009). Regulation of p53--insights into a complex process. *Crit. Rev. Biochem. Mol. Biol.* 44 (6) 367-392.
[54] Sharpless NE, Ramsey MR, Balasubramanian P, Castrillon DH, DePinho RA (2004). The differential impact of p16(INK4a) or p19(ARF) deficiency on cell growth and tumorigenesis. *Oncogene* 23 (2) 379-385.
[55] Koh J, Enders GH, Dynlacht BD, Harlow E (1995). Tumour-derived p16 alleles encoding proteins defective in cell-cycle inhibition. *Nature*, 375 (6531) 506-510.
[56] Baylin SB, Herman JG, Graff JR, Vertino PM, Issa JP (1998). Alterations in DNA methylation: a fundamental aspect of neoplasia. Adv *Cancer Res.* 72141-196.
[57] Forbes S, Clements J, Dawson E, Bamford S, Webb T, Dogan A, Flanagan A et al. (2006). Cosmic 2005. *Br. J. Cancer,* 94 (2) 318-322.
[58] Greenblatt MS, Beaudet JG, Gump JR, Godin KS, Trombley L, Koh J, Bond JP (2003). Detailed computational study of p53 and p16: using evolutionary sequence analysis and disease-associated mutations to predict the functional consequences of allelic variants. *Oncogene,* 22 (8) 1150-1163.
[59] Esteller M, Corn PG, Baylin SB, Herman JG (2001). A gene hypermethylation profile of human cancer. *Cancer Res.* 61 (8) 3225-3229.
[60] Arap W, Nishikawa R, Furnari FB, Cavenee WK, Huang HJ (1995). Replacement of the p16/CDKN2 gene suppresses human glioma cell growth. *Cancer Res.*55 (6) 1351-1354.
[61] Jin X, Nguyen D, Zhang WW, Kyritsis AP, Roth JA (1995). Cell cycle arrest and inhibition of tumor cell proliferation by the p16INK4 gene mediated by an adenovirus vector. *Cancer Res.* 55 (15) 3250-3253.
[62] Schrump DS, Chen GA, Consuli U, Jin X, Roth JA (1996). Inhibition of esophageal cancer proliferation by adenovirally mediated delivery of p16INK4. *Cancer Gene Ther.* 3 (6) 357-364.
[63] Campbell I, Magliocco A, Moyana T, Zheng C, Xiang J (2000). Adenovirus-mediated p16INK4 gene transfer significantly suppresses human breast cancer growth. *Cancer Gene Ther.* 7 (9) 1270-1278.
[64] Agarwal P, Sandey M, DeInnocentes P, Bird RC (2012). Tumor Suppressor Gene p16/INK4A/CDKN2A Dependent Regulation Into and Out of the Cell Cycle in a Spontaneous Canine Model of Breast Cancer. *J. Cell Biochem.* Manuscript in press.
[65] van 't Veer LJ, Dai H, van de Vijver MJ, He YD, Hart AA, Mao M, Peterse HL et al. (2002). Gene expression profiling predicts clinical outcome of breast cancer. *Nature* 415 (6871) 530-536.

[66] Saal LH, Johansson P, Holm K, Gruvberger-Saal SK, She QB, Maurer M, Koujak S et al. (2007). Poor prognosis in carcinoma is associated with a gene expression signature of aberrant PTEN tumor suppressor pathway activity. *Proc. Natl. Acad. Sci. U S A* 104 (18) 7564-7569.

[67] Wood LD, Parsons DW, Jones S, Lin J, Sjoblom T, Leary RJ, Shen D et al. (2007). The genomic landscapes of human breast and colorectal cancers. *Science* 318 (5853) 1108-1113.

[68] Ressel L, Millanta F, Caleri E, Innocenti VM, Poli A (2009). Reduced PTEN protein expression and its prognostic implications in canine and feline mammary tumors. *Vet. Pathol.* 46 (5) 860-868.

[69] Sweet-Cordero A, Mukherjee S, Subramanian A, You H, Roix JJ, Ladd-Acosta C, Mesirov J et al. (2005). An oncogenic KRAS2 expression signature identified by cross-species gene-expression analysis. *Nat. Genet.* 37 (1) 48-55.

[70] Sebolt-Leopold JS, Herrera R (2004). Targeting the mitogen-activated protein kinase cascade to treat cancer. *Nat. Rev. Cancer,* 4 (12) 937-947.

[71] Cadigan KM, Nusse R (1997). Wnt signaling: a common theme in animal development. *Genes Dev.* 11 (24) 3286-3305.

[72] Klaus A, Birchmeier W (2008). Wnt signalling and its impact on development and cancer. *Nat. Rev. Cancer,* 8 (5) 387-398.

[73] Suzuki H, Toyota M, Carraway H, Gabrielson E, Ohmura T, Fujikane T, Nishikawa N et al. (2008). Frequent epigenetic inactivation of Wnt antagonist genes in breast cancer. *Br. J. Cancer,*98 (6) 1147-1156.

[74] Rao NA, van Wolferen ME, van den Ham R, van Leenen D, Groot Koerkamp MJ, Holstege FC, Mol JA (2008). cDNA microarray profiles of canine mammary tumour cell lines reveal deregulated pathways pertaining to their phenotype. *Anim. Genet.* 39 (4) 333-345.

[75] Lagos-Quintana M, Rauhut R, Lendeckel W, Tuschl T (2001). Identification of novel genes coding for small expressed RNAs. *Science* 294 (5543) 853-858.

[76] Esquela-Kerscher A, Slack FJ (2006). Oncomirs - microRNAs with a role in cancer. *Nat. Rev. Cancer,* 6 (4) 259-269.

[77] Calin GA, Sevignani C, Dumitru CD, Hyslop T, Noch E, Yendamuri S, Shimizu M et al. (2004). Human microRNA genes are frequently located at fragile sites and genomic regions involved in cancers. *Proc. Natl. Acad. Sci. U S A* 101 (9) 2999-3004.

[78] Iorio MV, Ferracin M, Liu CG, Veronese A, Spizzo R, Sabbioni S, Magri E et al. (2005). MicroRNA gene expression deregulation in human breast cancer. *Cancer Res.* 65 (16) 7065-7070.

[79] Qi L, Bart J, Tan LP, Platteel I, Sluis T, Huitema S, Harms G et al. (2009). Expression of miR-21 and its targets (PTEN, PDCD4, TM1) in flat epithelial atypia of the breast in relation to ductal carcinoma in situ and invasive carcinoma. *BMC Cancer*, 9163.

[80] Zhu S, Si ML, Wu H, Mo YY (2007). MicroRNA-21 targets the tumor suppressor gene tropomyosin 1 (TPM1). *J. Biol. Chem.* 282 (19) 14328-14336.

[81] Frankel LB, Christoffersen NR, Jacobsen A, Lindow M, Krogh A, Lund AH (2008). Programmed cell death 4 (PDCD4) is an important functional target of the microRNA miR-21 in breast cancer cells. *J. Biol. Chem.* 283 (2) 1026-1033.

[82] Zhu S, Wu H, Wu F, Nie D, Sheng S, Mo YY (2008). MicroRNA-21 targets tumor suppressor genes in invasion and metastasis. *Cell Res.* 18 (3) 350-359.

[83] Si ML, Zhu S, Wu H, Lu Z, Wu F, Mo YY (2007). miR-21-mediated tumor growth. *Oncogene* 26 (19) 2799-2803.

[84] Boggs RM, Wright ZM, Stickney MJ, Porter WW, Murphy KE (2008). MicroRNA expression in canine mammary cancer. *Mamm. Genome* 19 (7-8) 561-569.

[85] American Cancer Society (2011). Cancer Facts and Figures 2011. Atlanta, GA: American Cancer Society.

[86] Shankland KR, Armitage JO, Hancock BW (2012). Non-Hodgkin lymphoma. *Lancet* 380 (9844) 848-857.

[87] Vail DM, Young KM (2007). Hematopoietic tumors: Canine lymphoma and lymphoid leukemia. In: Withrow SJ, Vail DM (eds) Small Animal Clinical Oncology, (p699), Philadelphia, W.B. Saunders.

[88] Modiano JF, Breen M, Valli VE, Wojcieszyn JW, Cutter GR (2007). Predictive value of p16 or Rb inactivation in a model of naturally occurring canine non-Hodgkin's lymphoma. *Leukemia* 21 (1) 184-187.

[89] Morton LM, Wang SS, Devesa SS, Hartge P, Weisenburger DD, Linet MS (2006). Lymphoma incidence patterns by WHO subtype in the United States, 1992-2001. *Blood* 107 (1) 265-276.

[90] Modiano JF, Breen M, Burnett RC, Parker HG, Inusah S, Thomas R, Avery PR et al. (2005). Distinct B-cell and T-cell lymphoproliferative disease prevalence among dog breeds indicates heritable risk. *Cancer Res.* 65 (13) 5654-5661.

[91] Pastor M, Chalvet-Monfray K, Marchal T, Keck G, Magnol JP, Fournel-Fleury C, Ponce F (2009). Genetic and environmental risk indicators in canine non-Hodgkin's lymphomas: breed associations and geographic distribution of 608 cases diagnosed throughout France over 1 year. *J. Vet. Intern Med.*23 (2) 301-310.

[92] Thomas R, Seiser EL, Motsinger-Reif A, Borst L, Valli VE, Kelley K, Suter SE et al. (2011). Refining tumor-associated aneuploidy through 'genomic recoding' of recurrent DNA copy number aberrations in 150 canine non-Hodgkin lymphomas. *Leuk. Lymphoma,* 52 (7) 1321-1335.

[93] Higgins RA, Blankenship JE, Kinney MC (2008). Application of immuno-histochemistry in the diagnosis of non-Hodgkin and Hodgkin lymphoma. *Arch. Pathol. Lab. Med.* 132 (3) 441-461.

[94] Valli VE, San Myint M, Barthel A, Bienzle D, Caswell J, Colbatzky F, Durham A et al. (2011). Classification of canine malignant lymphomas according to the World Health Organization criteria. *Vet. Pathol.* 48 (1) 198-211.

[95] O'Connor R (2007). The pharmacology of cancer resistance. *Anticancer Res.* 27 (3A) 1267-1272.

[96] Bergman PJ, Ogilvie GK, Powers BE (1996). Monoclonal antibody C219 immuno-histochemistry against P-glycoprotein: sequential analysis and predictive ability in dogs with lymphoma. *J. Vet. Intern Med.* 10 (6) 354-359.

[97] Lee JJ, Hughes CS, Fine RL, Page RL (1996). P-glycoprotein expression in canine lymphoma: a relevant, intermediate model of multidrug resistance. *Cancer* 77 (9) 1892-1898.

[98] Moore AS, Leveille CR, Reimann KA, Shu H, Arias IM (1995). The expression of P-glycoprotein in canine lymphoma and its association with multidrug resistance. *Cancer Investigation.* 13 (5) 475-479.

[99] Tomiyasu H, Goto-Koshino Y, Takahashi M, Fujino Y, Ohno K, Tsujimoto H (2010). Quantitative analysis of mRNA for 10 different drug resistance factors in dogs with lymphoma. *J. Vet. Med. Sci.* 72 (9) 1165-1172.

[100] Ferry JA (2006). Burkitt's lymphoma: clinicopathologic features and differential diagnosis. *Oncologist*, 11 (4) 375-383.

[101] Hahn KA, Richardson RC, Hahn EA, Chrisman CL (1994). Diagnostic and prognostic importance of chromosomal aberrations identified in 61 dogs with lymphosarcoma. *Vet. Pathol.* 31 (5) 528-540.

[102] Thomas R, Smith KC, Ostrander EA, Galibert F, Breen M (2003). Chromosome aberrations in canine multicentric lymphomas detected with comparative genomic hybridisation and a panel of single locus probes. *Br. J. Cancer,* 89 (8) 1530-1537.

[103] Marconato L, Gelain ME, Comazzi S (2012). The dog as a possible animal model for human non-Hodgkin lymphoma: a review. *Hematol. Oncol.*

[104] Lawrie CH (2008). MicroRNA expression in lymphoid malignancies: new hope for diagnosis and therapy? *J. Cell Mol. Med.* 12 (5A) 1432-1444.

[105] Uhl E, Krimer P, Schliekelman P, Tompkins SM, Suter S (2011). Identification of altered MicroRNA expression in canine lymphoid cell lines and cases of B- and T-Cell lymphomas. *Genes Chromosomes Cancer* 50 (11) 950-967.

[106] Mortarino M, Gioia G, Gelain ME, Albonico F, Roccabianca P, Ferri E, Comazzi S (2010). Identification of suitable endogenous controls and differentially expressed microRNAs in canine fresh-frozen and FFPE lymphoma samples. *Leuk. Res.* 34 (8) 1070-1077.

[107] Wheeler DA, Srinivasan M, Egholm M, Shen Y, Chen L, McGuire A, He W et al. (2008). The complete genome of an individual by massively parallel DNA sequencing. *Nature* 452 (7189) 872-876.

[108] Rosa-Rosa JM, Gracia-Aznarez FJ, Hodges E, Pita G, Rooks M, Xuan Z, Bhattacharjee A et al. (2010). Deep sequencing of target linkage assay-identified regions in familial breast cancer: methods, analysis pipeline and troubleshooting. *PLoS One* 5 (4) e9976.

[109] Kim RN, Kim DS, Choi SH, Yoon BH, Kang A, Nam SH, Kim DW et al. (2012). Genome analysis of the domestic dog (Korean Jindo) by massively parallel sequencing. *DNA Res.* 19 (3) 275-287.

In: Animal Models in Cancer Research ...
Editor: Sean A. Murray

ISBN: 978-1-62417-587-9

Chapter IV

Development of Cell Therapeutic Strategies for Alzheimer's Disease Using Animal Models

Kazuyuki Takata**, Shohei Kawanishi, Yumiko Touji, Tetsuya Takada, Yoshihisa Kitamura and Eishi Ashihara
Department of Clinical and Translational Physiology,
Kyoto Pharmaceutical University, Misasagi, Yamashina-ku, Kyoto, Japan

Abstract

Alzheimer's disease (AD) is characterized by progressive cognitive impairment as a consequence of extensive neuronal loss. Pathological hallmarks of AD include the development of senile plaques formed by the accumulation of extracellular amyloid-β(Aβ) and neurofibrillary tangles (NFTs) consisting of intraneuronal accumulation of hyperphosphorylated tau. According to the amyloid cascade hypothesis, the accumulation of Aβin the brain parenchyma is the early event that influences other AD pathologies. Therefore, the reduction of brain Aβhas been considered a primary therapeutic target for AD. Since familial AD-linked genes have been found, many transgenic mouse models have been established and utilized in the experimental studies to examine the accuracy of amyloid cascade hypothesis and therapeutic strategies. In the studies, microglial phagocytosis has been noted as an Aβclearance system in the brain. Interestingly, microglia exogenously administered also affect the clearance of Aβ. In this context, cell therapeutic strategies aiming at replenishment of microglia-dependent functions in the brain have been proposed and the feasibility is about to be examined in the experimental study using transgenic mouse models of AD. In this chapter, we focused on cell therapeutic strategies, which have been constructed by the microglial beneficial functions, then summarized the current status of the studies. Experimental evidence hopefullysuggest that the cell-based therapeutic approach could be a powerful strategy for AD treatment.

---

* Corresponding author: KazuyukiTakata, Ph.D. Department of Clinical and Translational Physiology, Kyoto Pharmaceutical University, Kyoto 607–8414, Japan; TEL: +81(Japan)–75–595–4706; FAX: +81(Japan)–75–595–4796; E–mail address: kaz@mb.kyoto-phu.ac.jp.

Introduction

Alzheimer's disease (AD) is the most common cause of dementia and the principal risk factor is aging. AD treatments currently approved are commonly regarded as purely symptomatic, and there is no disease-modifying treatment for AD. Therefore, the more effective therapies based on AD pathologies are eagerly required by prospects for increasing prevalence due to population aging all over the world. Neuropathological hallmarks of AD are extracellular amyloid depositions (senile plaques) and intracellular neurofibrillary tangles (NFTs) along with extensive neuronal loss [1]. Senile plaques consist of amyloid-β (Aβ) peptides that are surrounded by dystrophic neurites and reactive glial cells [2]. Aβ is derived from the sequential proteolysis of amyloid precursor protein (APP) by β- and γ-secretases. NFTs are formed by the abnormal intraneuronal aggregation of hyper-phosphorylated tau proteins [3]. Although most cases of AD occur sporadically and are not genetically inherited, small populations of patients develop autosomal dominant AD (familial AD) [4]. In the studies of familial AD, mutations in genes of *APP* on chromosome 21, *presenilin(PS) 1* gene on chromosome 14, and *PS2* gene on chromosome 1 have been found. The discovery of familial AD-linked mutant genes has allowed the creation of transgenic mouse models for AD, and all mutations overexpressed in transgenic mice enhance the Aβ production in the brain. This fact critically contributes to the establishment of "amyloid cascade hypothesis" that indicates the accumulation of Aβ in brains is the primary event driving AD development [5]. To demonstrate the integrity of the amyloid cascade hypothesis and to investigate novel therapeutic strategies for AD, further studies using the transgenic mouse models of AD are continuing. Pre-clinical studies of Aβ immunotherapy represent the discovery of novel therapeutic strategies for AD. Immunization with Aβ peptide in transgenic mouse models of AD significantly reduced the formation and deposition of Aβ in the brain and restored cognitive function [6-9]. In the studies, microglial Aβphagocytosis has been proposed as a principal mechanism for Aβ clearance in the brain [10]. Microglia are the primary immune effector cells distributed ubiquitously throughout the central nervous system (CNS), and play a role in the surveillance and repair of CNS. Recently, it was suggested that age-related microglial dystrophy and senescence may occur to a greater extent in neuro-degenerative conditions and may be a risk factor in AD development [11, 12]. Therefore, the recruitment and replenishment of newly differentiated microglia and/or microglia-like monocytic cells from hematopoietic stem cells (HSCs) in peripheral blood and bone marrow (BM) are thought to be a new therapeutic strategy. In this chapter, the latest findings regarding the cell therapeutic approach in AD, using transgenic mouse models of AD, are summarized and the possibilities of developing a novel AD treatment are discussed.

Amyloid Cascade Hypothesis

The amyloid cascade hypothesis, which indicates the accumulation of Aβ in the brain, is the primary event driving other AD pathologies, such as NFTs formations, synaptic deficits and neuronal loss as the result from an imbalance between Aβ production and Aβ clearance, and offers a broad framework to explain AD pathogenesis [5]. Aβ peptides are produced from APP by combination cleavages with β-secretase and γ-secretase and is composed of 37–43 amino acid residues because γ-secretase, which is a protein complex including PS, generates the C-terminal of Aβ with different lengths [13]. The major species of Aβ detected in the AD brain are Aβ1-40 (Aβ40) and Aβ1-42 (Aβ42). Aβ42 is prone to aggregation [14], indicates more neurotoxicity than Aβ40 [15], and predominantly consists of Aβ plaques [16]. On the other hand, Aβ40 is the major soluble species and is secreted 10-fold more than Aβ42 in normal brains. In the AD brain, a previous study demonstrated that the deposition of Aβ40 particularly correlated with synaptic and neuronal loss [17]. Furthermore, the potent fibrillization and neurotoxicity of Aβ1-43 (Aβ43)has been recently reported [18]. On the initial establishment of amyloid cascade hypothesis, investigations into the temporal changes in Down's syndrome pathologies were significantly referenced. Down's syndrome (Trisomy 21), which invariably shows the neuropathology of AD, the *APP* gene on the chromosome 21 is 1.5-fold and the formation of Aβ plaques precedes other AD-specific neuropathologies and cognitive impairment [19, 20]. Subsequently, familial AD-linked gene mutations were found on three genes, namely *APP*, *PS1*, and *PS2*, and it was revealed that all mutations are involved in the promotion of Aβ production. In this process, transgenic mouse models of AD harboring the familial AD-linked mutant genes were generated for the first time and critically contributed to the establishment of the amyloid cascade hypothesis. In addition, production and clearance rate of Aβ in *in vivo* human CNS was recently measured to be 7.6% per hour and 8.3% per hour, respectively [21], and a decreased clearance rate of Aβ has been reported in patients with late-onset "sporadic" AD, accounting for 99% of all AD cases [22]. Therefore, the dysregulation of Aβ clearance seems to be critically involved in the sporadic AD pathogenesis, and this evidence further emphasizes the integrity of the amyloid cascade hypothesis.

Transgenic Mice Models of AD

So far, numerous transgenic mouse models of AD have been created by the transgenes of familial AD-linked mutant genes. In this chapter, we focus on important prototypes in each class and models that are most commonly used (Table 1). The first transgenic mice model, termed PDAPP mice, which recapitulated AD pathologies, was generated by the over-expression of a human APP containing the Indiana mutation (V717F), a mutation found in familial AD, under the control of the platelet-derived growth factor-β (PDGF-β) promoter [23]. The transgenic mice promoted the Aβ production and recapitulated age-related extra-cellular Aβ depositions associated with dystrophic neurites and gliosis that began at approximately 8 months. The mice further showed synaptic loss and deficits of spatial learning and memory except for the overt neuronal loss [24, 25]. The most widely utilized AD transgenic mouse model has been Tg2576 mice [26]. Tg2576 mice overexpress a human APP containing the familial AD-linked Swedish mutation (K670N/M671L) driven by a hamster prion protein promoter and exhibit an age-dependent increase of Aβ40 and Aβ42 resulting in Aβ depositions at 9-13 months of age. Although Aβ deposits were associated with dystrophic neurites and activated glial cells, overt neuronal loss was not detected in Tg2576 mice, likewise PDAPP mice [27]. Tg2576 mice also exhibit impaired spatial learning and memory [28, 29].

Table 1. Representative transgenic mouse models of AD

Mouse Model	Transgene	Promoter	Aβ plaques formation (month)	NFTs-like lesion (month)	Cognitive impairment (month)	Reference Number
PDAPP	APP (V717F)	PDGF-β	6-9	No	6	6, 9, 10, 23, 24, 25, 47
Tg2576	APP (K670N/M671L)	PrP	9	No	10	26, 27, 28, 29
PS1	PS1 (M146L)	PDGF-β	No	No	No	30
PS/APP	APP (K670N/M671L) PS1 (M146L)	PrP PDGF-β	6	No	4	8, 32, 86
APPPS1	APP (K670N/M671L) PS1 (L166P)	Thy-1 Thy-1	1.5-2	No	8	48, 49
APdE9	APP (K670N/M671L) PS1 (exon 9-deleted)	PrP PrP	6	No	6	63, 64, 82 88
PSswe/ PS1	APP (K670N/M671L) PS1 (A246E)	PrP PrP	9-12	No	6	81, 83, 86
JNPL3	Tau (P301L)	PrP	No	4.5-6.5	motor deficits	33
TAPP	APP (K670N/M671L) Tau (P301L)	PrP PrP	8-15	3-6	motor deficits	34
3xTg-AD	APP (K670N/M671L) Tau (P301L) PS1 (M146L)	Thy-1 Thy-1 PS1	6	12-18	4.5	35, 36, 37

APP: amyloid precursor protein, PS1: presenilin 1, PDGF-β: platelet-derived growth factor-β, PrP: prion protein, Thy-1: thymocyte differentiation antigen-1.

Subsequently, many lines of transgenic mice were developed by the overexpression of *APP* genes containing single or multiple familial AD-linked mutations with various promoters. In general, these lines develop robust amyloid pathology and have synaptic damage and memory deficits but do not typically exhibit NFTs formation and significant neuronal loss.

The most common autosomal dominant AD-linked gene mutations have been found on the*PS1* gene. The mutations of *PS1* genes have been used to make mouse models of AD. In transgenic mice, named PS1 mice, overexpression of mutant PS1 (M146L) with a PDGF-βpromoter, increases Aβ42 production with no effect on Aβ40 levels in the brains [30]. However, PS1 mice do not develop Aβ depositions or cognitive deficits probably due to the differences of amino acid sequence in APP and Aβ between mouse and human [31];the mutation ofPS1 significantly accelerate the Aβ depositions induced by the overexpression of human mutant APP. Tg2576 mice and PS1 mice were crossed to generate the double transgenic PS/APP line, which express human APP with Swedish mutation and mutant PS1 (M146L) [32]. PS/APP mice show a selective increase of Aβ42 production and develop large numbers of fibrillarAβ plaques earlier than Tg2576 mice. Thus, many transgenic mouse models of AD have been established by transgenes of familialAD-linked mutation, and the transgenic mice have clearly exhibited that all mutations are related to the promotion of Aβ production.

NFTs-like neuronal lesions were first recapitulated by the transgenic mice, known as JNPL3 mice, which express the human mutant tau (P301L) found in frontotemporal dementia and Parkinsonism linked to chromosome 17 (FTDP-17) [33]. It is important to note that tau mutations do not cause AD, and thus it is unclear that the mechanism induced by tau mutations is involved in AD pathophysiologies. However, informative evidence, which shows the relationship between pathologies of Aβ and tau, has been found in the transgenic mice overexpressing both human mutant APP and human mutant tau. The original transgenic mice harboring double mutations of APP and tau, called TAPP mice, were established by crossing Tg2576 mice and JNPL3 mice [34]. The TAPP mice undergo increased formation of hyperphosphorylatedtau-positive NFTs-like lesion as compared with JNPL3 mice, whereas the structure and number of their Aβ plaques are essentially unaltered against those formed in Tg2576 mice. Later, a triple transgenic mouse model of AD, termed 3xTg-AD mice, was generated by co-injection of human APP with Swedish mutation and human tau with the P301L mutation into embryonic cells expressing human mutant PS1 (M146V). The 3xTg-AD mice develop extracellular Aβ deposits before NFTs-like neuronal pathology [35]. In the study on 3xTg-AD mice, we further found that Aβ links NFTs pathology and synaptic pathologies through the intraneuronal accumulation of Wiskott-Aldrich syndrome protein family verprolin-homologousprotein (WAVE), a key molecule for actin assembly [36]. Although the WAVE accumulation was also found in the NFTs of the AD brain, we did not find it in brains of JNPL3 mice, which develop NFTs-like pathology alone without Aβ accumulation. Taken together, these findings suggest that altered APP processing and Aβ production occurs before the tau alterations and exacerbate NFTs pathology. Thus, evidence in the transgenic mouse models of AD strongly supports the amyloid cascade hypothesis. Thus, transgenic mice are models for familial AD rather than sporadic AD, accounting for 99% of all AD cases, and there is no animal model that individually recapitulates all pathologies developed in AD. However, the construction of the transgenic mouse models by transgenes of familial AD-linked mutations has provided deep insight into the pathophysiology of AD. Based on the evidence, therapeutic approaches have been considered using transgenic mouse models of AD.

Therapeutic Strategies Using Transgenic Mice Models of AD

Since the establishment of transgenic mouse models of AD, a number of experimental studies have been examined to provide novel therapeutic strategies for AD together with the confirmation on the integrity of amyloid cascade hypothesis. The representative studies are examination of Aβ immunotherapy. Immunization with Aβ peptide or administration of anti-Aβ antibodies in transgenic mouse models of AD, such as PDAPP mice, significantly reduced the formation and deposition of Aβ and restored cognitive function [6-10]. Furthermore, Aβ immunization in 3xTg-AD mice, which develop Aβ plaque and NFTs-like pathologies, resulted in reduced levels of not only Aβ but also hyperphosphorylated tau [37]. Several mechanisms of Aβ clearance have been proposed, such as Fc-receptor-mediated microglial phagocytosis [10], drainage of soluble brain Aβ into the plasma [38], and antibody-mediated disaggregation of amyloid fibrils [39]. Subsequently, based on studies in mice, a clinical trial of an active Aβ vaccine (AN1792) subjected to human AD patients was performed. Unfortunately, 18 of 298 (6%) patients treated with AN1792 showed signs of developing encephalitis and/or meningoencephalitis so the trial was halted in 2002 [40, 41]. However, in a case report of the clinical trial, phagocytic microglia were found in the brain area that was devoid of Aβ, and microglial contribution of the Aβ clearance in the AD brain was suggested [42]. Thus, microglial Aβphagocytosis is thought to be at least one mechanism of Aβ clearance in the brain.

Microglia in the AD Brain

Microglia are distributed ubiquitously throughout CNS and are thought to make up approximately5% of the entire cell population in the cerebral cortex [43]. In the brain, microglia are considered to be a sensor to survey the CNS microenvironment with highly branched and motile processes under the physiological condition [44, 45].

Under the neurodegenerative conditions induced by trauma, infections, ischemia, and other diseases, microglia dramatically change its morphology from branched form (ramified form) to swollen and round forms (busy and ameboid forms) and accumulate on the damaged area to develop various immune reactions, such as phagocytosis and cytokine productions [46]. Activation of microglia has been believed to lead to neurotoxic effect because of results of *in vitro* culture studies, which reflects only one possible phenotype of microglia. However, recent studies of the *in vivo* brain revealed that microglia participate in defense processes of the brain.

Therefore, much attention has been given to beneficial functions of microglia with the viewpoint of a therapeutic approach to neurodegenerative diseases.

In the brain of patients with AD, it is well known that the activated microglia accumulate on the Aβ deposits [2]. The accumulation of microglia was initially postulated to be involved in the formation of Aβ depositions in the brain [41]. However, recent *in vivo* multiphoton microscopic studies clearly demonstrated that microglia rapidly migrate toward the Aβ depositions after the Aβ plaque formation in the brains of transgenic mice overexpressing green fluorescent protein (GFP) in microglia crossed with PDAPP mice [47] or APPPS1 mice expressing both APP with Swedish mutation and mutant PS1 (L166P) [48, 49].

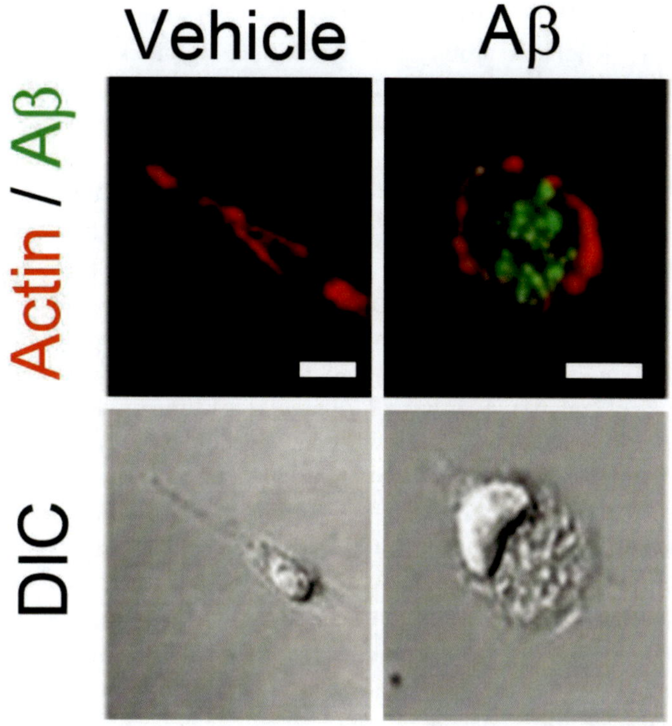

Figure 1. Aβ phagocytosis by primary cultured rat microglia. After the treatment of vehicle or Aβ, microglia were probed with rhodamine-phalloidin (for actin staining: red) and anti-Aβ antibody (green). Images are obtained by a confocal laser microscopy. Rat microglia changed its shape from a rod-like shape to an amoeboid shape, and then phagocytosed Aβ. Scale bars = 10 μm. DIC: differential interference contrast.

For the recognition of Aβ, microglia may utilize many cell surface receptors, such as scavenger receptors [50-53], receptor complexes comprising CD36, α6β1 integrin, and CD47 [54, 55], and the receptor for advanced glycation end products (RAGE) [56], and furthermore, phagocytose Aβ. We previously investigated in detail the microglial Aβ phagocytosis using primary cultured rat microglia [57, 58]. After the treatment of Aβ42 peptide, microglia immediately changed its shape from a rod-like shape to an amoeboid shape, and then markedly phagocytosed Aβ [57] (Figure 1). This microglial Aβ phagocytosis was inhibited by the pre-incubation of cytochalasin D, an inhibitor of actin reorganization. After the microglial Aβ phagocytosis, we further demonstrated that the clearance of Aβ in microglia might be mediated by peptidases such as insulin-degrading enzyme (IDE)-like peptidases and/or cathepsin D-like protease [58]. Microglia also seem to phagocytose oligomeric Aβ, which is a more neurotoxic Aβ species [59], and degrade it with IDE and/or neprilysin (NEP) [60]. Taken together, microglia may have abilities to phagocytose and degrade Aβ peptides, and the cell surface receptors, reorganization of actin cytoskeleton, and several peptidases may play an important role in the Aβ phagocytosis and clearance. Thus, it is suggested that microglia accumulated on the Aβ plaques may beneficially contribute to the suppression of AD development by phagocytosis and clearance of Aβ in brains.

Despite the presence of abundant plaque-associated microglia in the brains of AD, microglia seems to fail to efficiently clear Aβ deposits. Streit *et al.* reported age-related microglial dystrophy, senescence [11, 12], and dysfunction of Aβ phagocytosis [61], and further speculated a possibility that microglial senescence may be exacerbated by the presence of Aβ [62]. Khoury's group also reported the age-dependent dysfunction of Aβ phagocytosis in the study using primary-cultured microglia isolated from an aged transgenic mouse model of AD, named APdE9 mice, which express human APP with Swedish mutation and mutant exon 9-deleted variant of human PS1 [63, 64]. In the study, authors found an age-dependent decrease in the expression of the Aβ-binding receptors, such as scavenger receptor A, CD36, and RAGE, and the Aβ-degrading enzymes, such as IDE and neprilysin. In the aged microglia, they also found an inverse correlation between Aβ phagocytosis and prion-flammatory cytokine production, such as interleukin-1β and tumor necrosis factor-α (TNF-α), and further demonstrated that proinflammatory cytokines downregulate the expression of scavenger receptor A and CD36 and decrease Aβ phagocytosis. In addition, an age-dependent phenotypic change of microglia from alternative activation state with Aβ phagocytic capabilities (younger stage) to a classic cytotoxic phenotype expressing proinflammatory cytokines (older stage) was demonstrated by Jimenez*et al.* using other transgenic PS1 x APP mice lines [65].

This switch seems to be induced by the age-dependent accumulation of extracellular soluble Aβ oligomers, and may exacerbate neurodegeneration. Thus, in AD brains, microglial dysfunction may be induced by senescence and/or Aβ, and it is further speculated that the advance of AD pathogenesis results from the decreased ability of Aβ clearance and the aberrant proinflammatory state in microglia. In this context, recruitment and replenishment of newly differentiated microglia and/or microglia-like monocytic cells from HSCs in peripheral blood and BM are thought to be a new therapeutic strategy.

Cell Therapeutic Strategies for AD

In an *ex vivo* experimental study using unfixed brain sections from both AD cases and PDAPP mice, Bard *et al.* demonstrated that exogenously administered microglia affect the clearance of Aβ by the phagocytosis [10]. These findings suggest the potential of exogenous microglia as a cell therapeutic approach in AD. Therefore, we prepared primary cultured microglia from brains of newborn rats labeled with super-paramagnetic iron particles for the trace of magnetic resonance imaging, and then injected them into the lateral ventricle of the Aβ-injected rat [66]. As the result, we found the migration of exogenous microglia tithe Aβ deposit and accelerated Aβ clearance in the brains of Aβ-injected rats. Thus, we demonstrated that the replenishment of exogenous microglia affects Aβ clearance in the *in vivo* brain. In the study, we directly administrated primary cultured microglia into the lateral ventricle. Other groups reported that intra-arterially injected microglia but not macrophages can migrate through an intact and/or injured BBB to the brain parenchyma using rodent ischemic models [67, 68]. Therefore, we speculate that the administration of exogenously prepared microglia from systemic circulation may be effective for the Aβ clearance in brain parenchyma, and this idea positively proposes cell therapeutic strategies for AD. However, in the clinical application of the cell therapeutic strategies for human AD, preparation of exogenous human microglia is a first and important step. Although ethical and technical difficulties preclude the preparation of the primary culture of human microglia, differentiation from stem cells, such as HSCs, to microglia could be a breakthrough.

Origin of microglia is uncertain and has been at the center of debate between two schools of thought: mesodermal orneuroectodermal. However, most of the many markers that recognize cell surface antigen of microglia cross-react with monocytes and macrophages. On the other hand, neuroectodermal markers, which recognize microglia, have not been revealed. Therefore, microglia are recently considered to originate from mesodermal (myeloid) monocyte/macrophage cell lineage because of similarities in cell surface molecular phenotype [69-71]. In the developing mouse brain, primitive amoeboid microglia were first observed in the yolk sac, which is one of the extra medullary sources of hematopoiesis, at embryonic day (E) 8 of the developing mouse brain, and these cells were distributed in the mesenchyme associated with the neuroepithelial basement membrane at E8.5[72]. The microglial progenitor cells are recruited from some routes in the developing central nervous system (CNS), such as parenchymal blood vessels, meninges, and the cerebroventricle zone since BBB formations are still immature [71, 73, 74]. Subsequently, microglial progenitor cells, which entered the brain parenchyma, then proliferate, migrate, and distribute throughout the developing brain. Thereafter, these cells transform into ramified microglia, and this cell type is the only population of microglial cell type in the brain from postnatal day 18[73].

In adulthood, it has been considered that microglial turnover occurs both by the proliferation of resident microglia and by the replenishment of progenitor cells from circulating blood or BM [43]. Indeed, recent studies using lethally irradiated green fluorescent protein (GFP) transgenic BM chimeric mouse, which parenchymal microglia retain the characteristics of the host, whereas peripheral blood cells are reconstituted by GFP-positive BM cells (BMCs), showed that BM-derived GFP-positive cells entered into the brain parenchyma, and differentiated into the microglia-like cells [75-79]. In the studies using transgenic mouse models of AD (APdE9 mice [63] and APPswe/PS1 mice [80, 81], respectively), Malm *et al.*[82] and Simard *et al.*[83] also showed that the BM-derived GFP-positive microglia-like cells migrate toward the Aβ plaques through the BBB. These studies suggest that microglial progenitor cells may be derived from HSCs exist in circulating blood or BM, and are able to migrate into the brain parenchyma through the BBB, and replenish resident microglia in the adult brain. It is worth mentioning that the microglial progenitors differentiate to microglia-like cells and accumulate on the Aβ depositions.

In addition, it was demonstrated that linage negative cells from mouse BM could be differentiated into microglia-like cells by the cultivation with primary mixed glial culture supplemented with macrophage-colony stimulating factor (M-CSF) in an *in vitro* study [84]. We further demonstrated that mice BMCs and human $CD34^+$ cells (HSCs), cultured with human M-CSF without primary cultured mixed glial cells, significantly express microglial markers, such as CD11b and/or ionized calcium binding adaptor molecule-1 and functionally-phagocytose Aβ peptides [85] (Figure 2). Taken together, two possibilities for the therapeutic strategies for AD are considered: (i) recruitment of endogenous microglial progenitor cells from circulating blood or BM into the brain parenchyma, and (ii) replenishment by the administration of exogenous microglia-like cells differentiated from HSCs corrected from peripheral blood and BM.

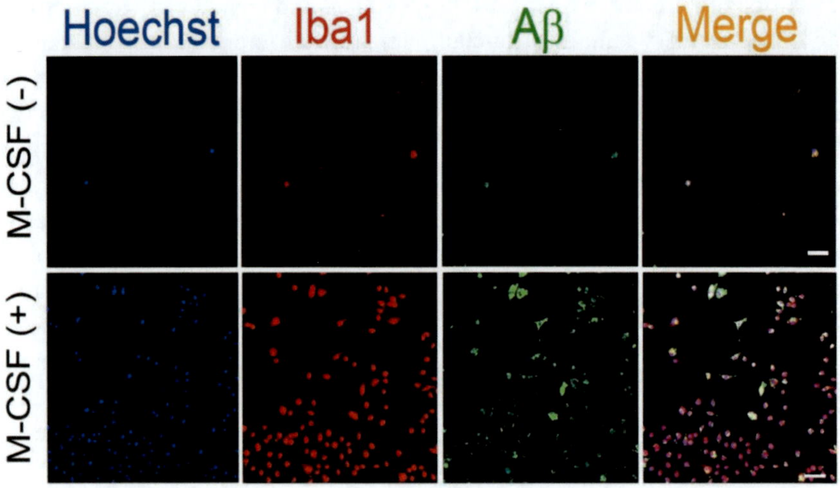

Figure 2. Aβ phagocytosis by mouse bone marrow-derived monocytic cells. Mouse bone marrow cells were cultivated for 7 days in the presence (+) or absence (-) of human M-CSF. Subsequently, cells were treated with Aβ. In the confocal laser microscopic analysis, cells were probed with Hoechst (for nuclei staining: blue) and antibodies against ionized calcium binding adaptor molecule-1 (Iba1, monocyte/microglia marker: red) and Aβ (green). Treatment of M-CSF markedly increased the numbers of total adherent cells (Hoechst), Iba1-possitive monocytic cells, and Aβ phagocytic cells. Scale bars = 50 μm.

Based on the former concept, Rivest's group demonstrated that chronic intraperitoneal administration of mouse M-CSF to APPswe/PS1 mice prevent cognitive loss, increase the number of microglia in the brain parenchyma, and decrease the number of Aβ plaques [86]. They also showed that the M-CSF treatment significantly increase the infiltration of GFP-positive cells into the brain parenchyma using APPswe/PS1-GFP chimeric mice of which peripheral blood cells are reconstituted by GFP-positive BMCs. Therefore, they suggested that chronic M-CSF treatment may increase the infiltration of BM-derived cells fated to be microglia-like cells into the brain parenchyma rather than the proliferation of resident microglia, and it promotes Aβ clearance and improves cognitive impairment in APPswe/PS1 mice. Thereafter, Bae's group intraperioneally injected human granulocyte colony stimulating factor (G-CSF) and AMD3000, an antagonist for CXCR4, to mobilize BM-derived HSCs into the blood, and further injected human stromal cell-derived factor-1α (SDF-1α), a strong chemo attractive factor for HSCs, into the hippocampus through the implanted guide cannula to promote the migration of the mobilized BM-derived HSCs into the brains of PS/APP mice [87]. With the treatments, they found improvement of memory deficit, increased microglial activation with neuroprotective phenotype and hippocampal neurogenesis, except for Aβ reduction. They also demonstrated that SDF-1α effectively induces the migration of GFP-labeled HSCs into the brain parenchyma using PS/APP-GFP chimeric mice. Therefore, they speculate that HSCs recruitment acts to improve cognitive function by modulating the inflammatory responses and activating a neuroprotective microglial phenotype, but does not affect Aβ clearance. Although the therapeutic mechanisms are still under debate between the two studies above, especially at the point of effectiveness on the Aβ clearance, the strategies of the recruitment of endogenous microglial progenitors from circulating blood or BM into the brain are hopefully expected to be developed as a novel treatment for AD.

Based on the latter concept, namely replenishment by the administration with exogenously prepared microglia-like cells, Koistinaho's group prepared monocytic cells derived from HSCs (mouse $CD117^+$ BM cells and human $CD34^+$ BM cells) by the treatment of M-CSF and transplanted the monocytic cells into the hippocampus of APdE9 mice [88]. In the study, they demonstrated that monocytic cells contribute to Aβ reduction in the brain. Although transplantation from the systemic circulation has not been examined yet, they speculated that monocytic cells obtained from human BM and mobilized peripheral blood HSCs could be potentially used for cell therapy for AD. Thus, transgenic mouse models of AD have been utilized for translational research in human AD therapy, and the studies hopefully suggest that the cell-based therapeutic approach could be a powerful strategy for AD treatment.

Conclusion

Since familial AD-linked genes are found, a lot of transgenic mouse models of AD are generated. Although no animal model individually recapitulates all pathologies developed in AD, studies using the mouse models have provided deep insights into the pathophysiology of AD and have critically contributed to the establishment of amyloid cascade hypothesis. Based on the evidence, the reduction of Aβ is considered a primary target on the therapeutic approaches for AD, and the role of microglia on AD pathologies attracted considerable attention due to its Aβ phagocytic ability. However, senescence and the dysfunctional state of residential microglia have been revealed in AD pathologies and are issued for therapeutic application. In this context, cell therapeutic strategies aiming at replenishment and restoration of microglia-dependent functions in the brain have been proposed. For this cell therapeutic approach, studies for the recruitment of endogenous microglial progenitor cells and administration of exogenous microglia-like cells have been started using transgenic mouse models of AD. Results hopefully suggested that the cell-based therapeutic approach could be a powerful strategy for AD treatment. Further studies are promised for the development of novel therapeutics for AD.

Acknowledgments

We thank Dr. Shun Shimohama, Department of Neurology, Sapporo Medical University, and Dr. IkuoTooyama, Molecular Neuroscience Research Center, Shiga University of Medical Science, for their collaboration in our studies referenced in this chapter. This chapter was supported by Ministry of Education, Culture, Sports, Science and Technology of Japan; grants–in–aid from Japan Society for the Promotion of Science; Takeda Science Foundation; SENSIN Medical Resarch Foundation; YOKOYAMA Foundation for Clinical Pharmacology;and Kyoto Pharmaceutical University Fund for the Promotion of Scientific Research.

References

[1] Selkoe, D. J. (1999). Translating cell biology into therapeutic advances in Alzheimer's disease. *Nature*, *399*, A23-31.

[2] Akiyama, H., Barger S., Barnum S., Bradt B., Bauer J., Cole G. M., et al. (2000). Inflammation and Alzheimer's disease. *Neurobiol. Aging*, *21*, 383-421.

[3] Ihara, Y., Nukina N., Miura R., Ogawara M. (1986). Phosphorylated tau protein is integrated into paired helical filaments in Alzheimer's disease. *J. Biochem.*, *99*, 1807-1810.

[4] Harvey, R. J., Skelton-Robinson M., Rossor M. N. (2003). The prevalence and causes of dementia in people under the age of 65 years. *J. Neurol. Neurosurg. Psychiatry*, *74*, 1206-1209.

[5] Hardy, J., Selkoe D. J. (2002). The amyloid hypothesis of Alzheimer's disease: progress and problems on the road to therapeutics. *Science*, *297*, 353-356.

[6] Dodart, J. C., Bales K. R., Gannon K. S., Greene S. J., DeMattos R. B., Mathis C., et al. (2002). Immunization reverses memory deficits without reducing brain Aβ burden in Alzheimer's disease model. *Nat. Neurosci.*, *5*, 452-457.

[7] Janus, C., Pearson J., McLaurin J., Mathews P. M., Jiang Y., Schmidt S. D., et al. (2000). Aβ peptide immunization reduces behavioural impairment and plaques in a model of Alzheimer's disease. *Nature*, *408*, 979-982.

[8] Morgan, D., Diamond D. M., Gottschall P. E., Ugen K. E., Dickey C., Hardy J., et al. (2000). Aβ peptide vaccination prevents memory loss in an animal model of Alzheimer's disease. *Nature*, *408*, 982-985.

[9] Schenk, D., Barbour R., Dunn W., Gordon G., Grajeda H., Guido T., et al. (1999). Immunization with amyloid-β attenuates Alzheimer-disease-like pathology in the PDAPP mouse. *Nature*, *400*, 173-177.

[10] Bard, F., Cannon C., Barbour R., Burke R. L., Games D., Grajeda H., et al. (2000). Peripherally administered antibodies against amyloid β-peptide enter the central nervous system and reduce pathology in a mouse model of Alzheimer disease. *Nat. Med.*, *6*, 916-919.

[11] Streit, W. J., Sammons N. W., Kuhns A. J., Sparks D. L. (2004). Dystrophic microglia in the aging human brain. *Glia*, *45*, 208-212.

[12] Flanary, B. E., Streit W. J. (2004). Progressive telomere shortening occurs in cultured rat microglia, but not astrocytes. *Glia*, *45*, 75-88.

[13] Wiltfang, J., Esselmann H., Bibl M., Smirnov A., Otto M., Paul S., et al. (2002). Highly conserved and disease-specific patterns of carboxyterminally truncated Aβ peptides 1-37/38/39 in addition to 1-40/42 in Alzheimer's disease and in patients with chronic neuroinflammation. *J. Neurochem.*, *81*, 481-496.

[14] Jarrett, J. T., Berger E. P., Lansbury P. T., Jr. (1993). The carboxy terminus of the β amyloid protein is critical for the seeding of amyloid formation: implications for the pathogenesis of Alzheimer's disease. *Biochemistry (Mosc).32*, 4693-4697.

[15] Dahlgren, K. N., Manelli A. M., Stine W. B., Jr., Baker L. K., Krafft G. A., LaDu M. J. (2002). Oligomeric and fibrillar species of amyloid-β peptides differentially affect neuronal viability. *J. Biol. Chem.*, *277*, 32046-32053.

[16] Iwatsubo, T., Odaka A., Suzuki N., Mizusawa H., Nukina N., Ihara Y. (1994). Visualization of Aβ 42(43) and Aβ 40 in senile plaques with end-specific Aβ monoclonals: evidence that an initially deposited species is Aβ 42(43). *Neuron*, *13*, 45-53.

[17] Lue, L. F., Kuo Y. M., Roher A. E., Brachova L., Shen Y., Sue L., et al. (1999). Soluble amyloid-β peptide concentration as a predictor of synaptic change in Alzheimer's disease. *Am. J. Pathol.*, *155*, 853-862.

[18] Saito, T., Suemoto T., Brouwers N., Sleegers K., Funamoto S., Mihira N., et al. (2011). Potent amyloidogenicity and pathogenicity of Abeta43. *Nat. Neurosci.*, *14*, 1023-1032.

[19] Mann, D. M., Esiri M. M. (1988). The site of the earliest lesions of Alzheimer's disease. *N. Engl. J. Med.*, *318*, 789-790.

[20] Mann, D. M. (1989). Cerebral amyloidosis, ageing and Alzheimer's disease; a contribution from studies on Down's syndrome. *Neurobiol. Aging*, *10*, 397-399; discussion 412-394.

[21] Bateman, R. J., Munsell L. Y., Morris J. C., Swarm R., Yarasheski K. E., Holtzman D. M. (2006). Human amyloid-beta synthesis and clearance rates as measured in cerebrospinal fluid in vivo. *Nat. Med.*, *12*, 856-861.

[22] Mawuenyega, K. G., Sigurdson W., Ovod V., Munsell L., Kasten T., Morris J. C., et al. (2010). Decreased clearance of CNS beta-amyloid in Alzheimer's disease. *Science*, *330*, 1774.

[23] Games, D., Adams D., Alessandrini R., Barbour R., Berthelette P., Blackwell C., et al. (1995). Alzheimer-type neuropathology in transgenic mice overexpressing V717F β-amyloid precursor protein. *Nature*, *373*, 523-527.

[24] Irizarry, M. C., Soriano F., McNamara M., Page K. J., Schenk D., Games D., et al. (1997). Abeta deposition is associated with neuropil changes, but not with overt neuronal loss in the human amyloid precursor protein V717F (PDAPP) transgenic mouse. *J. Neurosci.*, *17*, 7053-7059.

[25] Chen, G., Chen K. S., Knox J., Inglis J., Bernard A., Martin S. J., et al. (2000). A learning deficit related to age and beta-amyloid plaques in a mouse model of Alzheimer's disease. *Nature*, *408*, 975-979.

[26] Hsiao, K., Chapman P., Nilsen S., Eckman C., Harigaya Y., Younkin S., et al. (1996). Correlative memory deficits, Aβ elevation, and amyloid plaques in transgenic mice. *Science*, *274*, 99-102.

[27] Irizarry, M. C., McNamara M., Fedorchak K., Hsiao K., Hyman B. T. (1997). APPSw transgenic mice develop age-related A beta deposits and neuropil abnormalities, but no neuronal loss in CA1. *J. Neuropathol. Exp. Neurol.*, *56*, 965-973.

[28] Chapman, P. F., White G. L., Jones M. W., Cooper-Blacketer D., Marshall V. J., Irizarry M., et al. (1999). Impaired synaptic plasticity and learning in aged amyloid precursor protein transgenic mice. *Nat. Neurosci.*, *2*, 271-276.

[29] Jacobsen, J. S., Wu C. C., Redwine J. M., Comery T. A., Arias R., Bowlby M., et al. (2006). Early-onset behavioral and synaptic deficits in a mouse model of Alzheimer's disease. *Proc. Natl. Acad. Sci. U. S. A.*, *103*, 5161-5166.

[30] Duff, K., Eckman C., Zehr C., Yu X., Prada C. M., Perez-tur J., et al. (1996). Increased amyloid-beta42(43) in brains of mice expressing mutant presenilin 1. *Nature*, *383*, 710-713.

[31] Holcomb, L. A., Gordon M. N., Jantzen P., Hsiao K., Duff K., Morgan D. (1999). Behavioral changes in transgenic mice expressing both amyloid precursor protein and presenilin-1 mutations: lack of association with amyloid deposits. *Behav. Genet.*, *29*, 177-185.

[32] Holcomb, L., Gordon M. N., McGowan E., Yu X., Benkovic S., Jantzen P., et al. (1998). Accelerated Alzheimer-type phenotype in transgenic mice carrying both mutant amyloid precursor protein and presenilin 1 transgenes. *Nat. Med.*, *4*, 97-100.

[33] Lewis, J., McGowan E., Rockwood J., Melrose H., Nacharaju P., Van Slegtenhorst M., et al. (2000). Neurofibrillary tangles, amyotrophy and progressive motor disturbance in mice expressing mutant (P301L) tau protein. *Nat. Genet.*, *25*, 402-405.

[34] Lewis, J., Dickson D. W., Lin W. L., Chisholm L., Corral A., Jones G., et al. (2001). Enhanced neurofibrillary degeneration in transgenic mice expressing mutant tau and APP. *Science*, *293*, 1487-1491.

[35] Oddo, S., Caccamo A., Shepherd J. D., Murphy M. P., Golde T. E., Kayed R., et al. (2003). Triple-transgenic model of Alzheimer's disease with plaques and tangles: intracellular Abeta and synaptic dysfunction. *Neuron*, *39*, 409-421.

[36] Takata, K., Kitamura Y., Nakata Y., Matsuoka Y., Tomimoto H., Taniguchi T., et al. (2009). Involvement of WAVE accumulation in Aβ/APP pathology-dependent tangle modification in Alzheimer's disease. *Am. J. Pathol.*, *175*, 17-24.

[37] Oddo, S., Billings L., Kesslak J. P., Cribbs D. H., LaFerla F. M. (2004). Abeta immunotherapy leads to clearance of early, but not late, hyperphosphorylated tau aggregates via the proteasome. *Neuron*, *43*, 321-332.

[38] DeMattos, R. B., Bales K. R., Cummins D. J., Paul S. M., Holtzman D. M. (2002). Brain to plasma amyloid-beta efflux: a measure of brain amyloid burden in a mouse model of Alzheimer's disease. *Science*, *295*, 2264-2267.

[39] Solomon, B., Koppel R., Frankel D., Hanan-Aharon E. (1997). Disaggregation of Alzheimer beta-amyloid by site-directed mAb. *Proc. Natl. Acad. Sci. U. S. A.*, *94*, 4109-4112.

[40] Mathews, P. M., Nixon R. A. (2003). Setback for an Alzheimer's disease vaccine: lessons learned. *Neurology*, *61*, 7-8.

[41] Orgogozo, J. M., Gilman S., Dartigues J. F., Laurent B., Puel M., Kirby L. C., et al. (2003). Subacute meningoencephalitis in a subset of patients with AD after Abeta42 immunization. *Neurology*, *61*, 46-54.

[42] Nicoll, J. A., Wilkinson D., Holmes C., Steart P., Markham H., Weller R. O. (2003). Neuropathology of human Alzheimer disease after immunization with amyloid-β peptide: a case report. *Nat. Med.*, *9*, 448-452.

[43] Lawson, L. J., Perry V. H., Dri P., Gordon S. (1990). Heterogeneity in the distribution and morphology of microglia in the normal adult mouse brain. *Neuroscience*, *39*, 151-170.

[44] Davalos, D., Grutzendler J., Yang G., Kim J. V., Zuo Y., Jung S., et al. (2005). ATP mediates rapid microglial response to local brain injury in vivo. *Nat. Neurosci.*, *8*, 752-758.

[45] Nimmerjahn, A., Kirchhoff F., Helmchen F. (2005). Resting microglial cells are highly dynamic surveillants of brain parenchyma in vivo. *Science*, *308*, 1314-1318.

[46] Kitamura, Y., Nomura Y. (2003). Stress proteins and glial functions: possible therapeutic targets for neurodegenerative disorders. *Pharmacol. Ther.*, *97*, 35-53.

[47] Meyer-Luehmann, M., Spires-Jones T. L., Prada C., Garcia-Alloza M., de Calignon A., Rozkalne A., et al. (2008). Rapid appearance and local toxicity of amyloid-beta plaques in a mouse model of Alzheimer's disease. *Nature*, *451*, 720-724.

[48] Radde, R., Bolmont T., Kaeser S. A., Coomaraswamy J., Lindau D., Stoltze L., et al. (2006). Abeta42-driven cerebral amyloidosis in transgenic mice reveals early and robust pathology. *EMBO reports*, *7*, 940-946.

[49] Bolmont, T., Haiss F., Eicke D., Radde R., Mathis C. A., Klunk W. E., et al. (2008). Dynamics of the microglial/amyloid interaction indicate a role in plaque maintenance. *J. Neurosci.*, *28*, 4283-4292.

[50] El Khoury, J., Hickman S. E., Thomas C. A., Cao L., Silverstein S. C., Loike J. D. (1996). Scavenger receptor-mediated adhesion of microglia to beta-amyloid fibrils. *Nature*, *382*, 716-719.

[51] Paresce, D. M., Chung H., Maxfield F. R. (1997). Slow degradation of aggregates of the Alzheimer's disease amyloid beta-protein by microglial cells. *J. Biol. Chem.*, *272*, 29390-29397.

[52] Paresce, D. M., Ghosh R. N., Maxfield F. R. (1996). Microglial cells internalize aggregates of the Alzheimer's disease amyloid beta-protein via a scavenger receptor. *Neuron*, *17*, 553-565.

[53] Wilkinson, K., El Khoury J. (2012). Microglial scavenger receptors and their roles in the pathogenesis of Alzheimer's disease. *Int. J. Alzheimers. Dis.*, *2012*, 489456.

[54] Bamberger, M. E., Harris M. E., McDonald D. R., Husemann J., Landreth G. E. (2003). A cell surface receptor complex for fibrillar beta-amyloid mediates microglial activation. *J. Neurosci.*, *23*, 2665-2674.

[55] Koenigsknecht, J., Landreth G. (2004). Microglial phagocytosis of fibrillar beta-amyloid through a beta1 integrin-dependent mechanism. *J. Neurosci.*, *24*, 9838-9846.

[56] Yan, S. D., Chen X., Fu J., Chen M., Zhu H., Roher A., et al. (1996). RAGE and amyloid-beta peptide neurotoxicity in Alzheimer's disease. *Nature*, *382*, 685-691.

[57] Kitamura, Y., Shibagaki K., Takata K., Tsuchiya D., Taniguchi T., Gebicke-Haerter P. J., et al. (2003). Involvement of Wiskott-Aldrich syndrome protein family verprolin-homologous protein (WAVE) and Rac1 in the phagocytosis of amyloid-β(1-42) in rat microglia. *J. Pharmacol. Sci.*, *92*, 115-123.

[58] Kakimura, J., Kitamura Y., Takata K., Umeki M., Suzuki S., Shibagaki K., et al. (2002). Microglial activation and amyloid-β clearance induced by exogenous heat-shock proteins. *FASEB J.*, *16*, 601-603.

[59] Walsh, D. M., Klyubin I., Fadeeva J. V., Cullen W. K., Anwyl R., Wolfe M. S., et al. (2002). Naturally secreted oligomers of amyloid beta protein potently inhibit hippocampal long-term potentiation in vivo. *Nature*, *416*, 535-539.

[60] Shimizu, E., Kawahara K., Kajizono M., Sawada M., Nakayama H. (2008). IL-4-induced selective clearance of oligomeric β-amyloid peptide(1-42) by rat primary type 2 microglia. *J. Immunol.*, *181*, 6503-6513.

[61] Njie, E. G., Boelen E., Stassen F. R., Steinbusch H. W., Borchelt D. R., Streit W. J. (2012). Ex vivo cultures of microglia from young and aged rodent brain reveal age-related changes in microglial function. *Neurobiol. Aging*, *33*, 195 e191-112.

[62] Flanary, B. E., Sammons N. W., Nguyen C., Walker D., Streit W. J. (2007). Evidence that aging and amyloid promote microglial cell senescence. *Rejuvenation Res.*, *10*, 61-74.

[63] Jankowsky, J. L., Fadale D. J., Anderson J., Xu G. M., Gonzales V., Jenkins N. A., et al. (2004). Mutant presenilins specifically elevate the levels of the 42 residue beta-amyloid peptide in vivo: evidence for augmentation of a 42-specific gamma secretase. *Hum. Mol. Genet.*, *13*, 159-170.
[64] Hickman, S. E., Allison E. K., El Khoury J. (2008). Microglial dysfunction and defective β-amyloid clearance pathways in aging Alzheimer's disease mice. *J. Neurosci.*, *28*, 8354-8360.
[65] Jimenez, S., Baglietto-Vargas D., Caballero C., Moreno-Gonzalez I., Torres M., Sanchez-Varo R., et al. (2008). Inflammatory response in the hippocampus of PS1M146L/APP751SL mouse model of Alzheimer's disease: age-dependent switch in the microglial phenotype from alternative to classic. *J. Neurosci.*, *28*, 11650-11661.
[66] Takata, K., Kitamura Y., Yanagisawa D., Morikawa S., Morita M., Inubushi T., et al. (2007). Microglial transplantation increases amyloid-β clearance in Alzheimer model rats. *FEBS Lett.*, *581*, 475-478.
[67] Hayashi, Y., Tomimatsu Y., Suzuki H., Yamada J., Wu Z., Yao H., et al. (2006). The intra-arterial injection of microglia protects hippocampal CA1 neurons against global ischemia-induced functional deficits in rats. *Neuroscience*, *142*, 87-96.
[68] Imai, F., Suzuki H., Oda J., Ninomiya T., Ono K., Sano H., et al. (2007). Neuroprotective effect of exogenous microglia in global brain ischemia. *J. Cereb. Blood Flow Metab.*, *27*, 488-500.
[69] Chan, W. Y., Kohsaka S., Rezaie P. (2007). The origin and cell lineage of microglia: new concepts. *Brain Res. Rev.*, *53*, 344-354.
[70] Streit, W. J. (2001). Microglia and macrophages in the developing CNS. *Neurotoxicology*, *22*, 619-624.
[71] Cuadros, M. A., Navascues J. (1998). The origin and differentiation of microglial cells during development. *Prog. Neurobiol.*, *56*, 173-189.
[72] Kaur, C., Hao A. J., Wu C. H., Ling E. A. (2001). Origin of microglia. *Microsc. Res. Tech.*, *54*, 2-9.
[73] Dalmau, I., Vela J. M., Gonzalez B., Finsen B., Castellano B. (2003). Dynamics of microglia in the developing rat brain. *J. Comp. Neurol.*, *458*, 144-157.
[74] Ling, E. A., Wong W. C. (1993). The origin and nature of ramified and amoeboid microglia: a historical review and current concepts. *Glia*, *7*, 9-18.
[75] Asheuer, M., Pflumio F., Benhamida S., Dubart-Kupperschmitt A., Fouquet F., Imai Y., et al. (2004). Human CD34+ cells differentiate into microglia and express recombinant therapeutic protein. *Proc. Natl. Acad. Sci. U. S. A.*, *101*, 3557-3562.
[76] Hess, D. C., Abe T., Hill W. D., Studdard A. M., Carothers J., Masuya M., et al. (2004). Hematopoietic origin of microglial and perivascular cells in brain. *Exp. Neurol.*, *186*, 134-144.
[77] Massengale, M., Wagers A. J., Vogel H., Weissman I. L. (2005). Hematopoietic cells maintain hematopoietic fates upon entering the brain. *J. Exp. Med.*, *201*, 1579-1589.
[78] Simard, A. R., Rivest S. (2004). Bone marrow stem cells have the ability to populate the entire central nervous system into fully differentiated parenchymal microglia. *FASEB J.*, *18*, 998-1000.
[79] Vallieres, L., Sawchenko P. E. (2003). Bone marrow-derived cells that populate the adult mouse brain preserve their hematopoietic identity. *J. Neurosci.*, *23*, 5197-5207.

[80] Borchelt, D. R., Thinakaran G., Eckman C. B., Lee M. K., Davenport F., Ratovitsky T., et al. (1996). Familial Alzheimer's disease-linked presenilin 1 variants elevate Abeta1-42/1-40 ratio in vitro and in vivo. *Neuron*, *17*, 1005-1013.

[81] Borchelt, D. R., Ratovitski T., van Lare J., Lee M. K., Gonzales V., Jenkins N. A., et al. (1997). Accelerated amyloid deposition in the brains of transgenic mice coexpressing mutant presenilin 1 and amyloid precursor proteins. *Neuron*, *19*, 939-945.

[82] Malm, T. M., Koistinaho M., Parepalo M., Vatanen T., Ooka A., Karlsson S., et al. (2005). Bone-marrow-derived cells contribute to the recruitment of microglial cells in response to beta-amyloid deposition in APP/PS1 double transgenic Alzheimer mice. *Neurobiol. Dis.*, *18*, 134-142.

[83] Simard, A. R., Soulet D., Gowing G., Julien J. P., Rivest S. (2006). Bone marrow-derived microglia play a critical role in restricting senile plaque formation in Alzheimer's disease. *Neuron*, *49*, 489-502.

[84] Noto, D., Takahashi K., Miyake S., Yamada M. (2010). In vitro differentiation of lineage-negative bone marrow cells into microglia-like cells. *Eur. J. Neurosci.*, *31*, 1155-1163.

[85] Takata, K., Takada T., Tatsuda H., Tsuruno T., Nishimura K., Shimohama S., et al. (2011). Preparation and characterization of microglia-like cells derived from rat, mouse, and human bone marrow cells for therapeutic strategy of Alzheimer's disease. *J. Addiction Res. Ther.*, *S5*, 1-5.

[86] Boissonneault, V., Filali M., Lessard M., Relton J., Wong G., Rivest S. (2009). Powerful beneficial effects of macrophage colony-stimulating factor on beta-amyloid deposition and cognitive impairment in Alzheimer's disease. *Brain*, *132*, 1078-1092.

[87] Shinjo, S. K., Bonfa E., de Falco Caparbo V., Pereira R. M. (2011). Low bone mass in juvenile onset sclerosis systemic: the possible role for 25-hydroxyvitamin D insufficiency. *Rheumatol. Int.*, *31*, 1075-1080.

[88] Magga, J., Savchenko E., Malm T., Rolova T., Pollari E., Valonen P., et al. (2012). Production of monocytic cells from bone marrow stem cells: therapeutic usage in Alzheimer's disease. *J. Cell. Mol. Med.*, *16*, 1060-1073.

In: Animal Models in Cancer Research …
Editor: Sean A. Murray
ISBN: 978-1-62417-587-9

Chapter V

Animal Models for Antineoplastic Chemotherapy-Induced Alopecia

Tongyu C. Wikramanayake[1], Sonal Choudhary[1], Lucia M. Mauro[2] and Joaquin J. Jimenez[1,*]
[1]Department of Dermatology and Cutaneous Surgery,
University of Miami Miller School of Medicine, Miami, Florida, US
[2]Biochemistry and Molecular Biology, University of Miami Miller School of Medicine,
Miami, Florida, US

Abstract

One of the most common and distressing side effects of cancer therapy is chemotherapy-induced alopecia (CIA). Approximately 65% of patients receiving anti-neoplastic therapies experience some degree of alopecia. The study of CIA had been hampered by the lack of suitable animal models; in this regard, the first animal models used to study CIA were impractical and difficult to extrapolate to the humans. In recent years, the development of the young rat models and the mouse model of CIA opened new avenues to the investigation and understanding of the mechanisms of CIA. However, there has been much controversy as to which model is more suitable to study the histopathology and molecular mechanisms of CIA. The young rat model has been employed due to the fact that 100% of the pelage hair follicles are in the growth phase during postnatal morphogenesis, therefore mimicking the human scalp where 90% of the hair follicles are undergoing anagen (active growth phase of the hair cycle) at any given time. In contrast, in the adult mouse and rat models, anagen synchronization needs to be induced by depilation or shaving to mimic the human scalp. These models have been extensively used in the search for protective agents against CIA. In this chapter, we will compare and contrast the different models and review the state-of-the-art findings in terms of animal models and protective agents.

[*] Corresponding Author.Dr Joaquin J. Jimenez, Department of Dermatology and Cutaneous Surgery, University of Miami Miller School of Medicine,1600 NW 10th Avenue, RMSB 2023 A, Miam,FL 33136, USA.E-mail: jjimenez@med.miami.edu.

Introduction

Chemotherapy-induced alopecia (CIA) has consistently been classified as one of the most distressing side effects of cancer therapy. Approximately 65% of patients receiving anti-neoplastic therapies experience some degree of alopecia (Trueb 2010). While it is a benign medical condition that is generally reversible, CIA has an enormous psychosocial impact on the lives of cancer patients undergoing or considering chemotherapy. Alopecia has been cited by 47-58% of women with cancer as the most distressing side effect of chemotherapy, and as many as 8% of women in one study were found to be at risk of avoiding treatment due to the possibility of hair loss (McGarvey *et al.* 2001; Trueb 2010). Whereas research has been successful in developing treatments for other side effects of chemotherapy, it has fallen short in finding effective prevention and treatment strategies for CIA. However, studies on recently developed animal models of CIA have been instrumental in increasing our understanding of the mechanisms underlying CIA as well as leading the way for promising clinical trials.

The Biology of the Hair Follicles (HFs)

In order to better understand CIA, it is necessary to consider the biology of the hair follicles (HFs). Histologically, the HF consists of three sections: the infundibulum, which extends from the surface of the skin to the duct of the sebaceous gland; the isthmus, which extends from the sebaceous gland duct to the insertion point of the arrectorpili muscle; and finally the inferior segment, which extends from this insertion point to the matrix base (Habif 2010). Within the inferior segment are rapidly proliferating matrix cells in the hair bulb, interspersed with melanocytes, which together produce the pigmented hair shaft (Paus & Cotsarelis 1999). The mitotic rate of the matrix cells is one of the highest of all the organs in the body, and thus chemotherapeutic agents that target rapidly dividing cancer cells can have significantly detrimental effects on the matrix cells (Habif 2010). At the base of the HF, within an invagination of the matrix and inner root sheath lies the dermal papilla, which contains specialized fibroblasts that control the number of matrix cells and thus the size of hair (Paus & Cotsarelis 1999). The HF itself is composed of a hair shaft surrounded by components of the inner root sheath (IRS), the companion layer and the outer root sheath (ORS) (Shimomura & Christiano 2010). The hair shaft, or the emergent portion of the follicle, is composed of a central medulla surrounded by a multicellular layer called the cortex, which is encased by flattened cells making up the cuticle (Shimomura & Christiano 2010). The IRS consists of three distinct cell layers, namely the IRS cuticle, Huxley's layer, and Henle's layer. The IRS is a gelatinous mass that protects and molds the growing hair within the isthmus and inferior segments of the follicle via its own keratinization beginning in Henle's layer (Cheng & Baylisss 2008; Habif 2010). Surrounding the IRS is the companion layer, which itself is surrounded by the ORS. Within the ORS, and near the insertion site of the arrectorpili muscle, are the cells of the bulge region. These cells respond to signals from the dermal papilla during follicular morphogenesis as well as at the onset of subsequent hair cycles to regenerate the lower portion of the HF, and are characterized as epithelial stem cells (Paus & Cotsarelis 1999; Habif 2010). The ORS also consists of melanocytes, Langerhans' cells, and Merkel cells (Paus & Cotsarelis 1999).

After morphogenesis, HFs continuously cycles through three phases: anagen (growth), catagen (involution), and telogen (rest). On the human scalp, approximately 90% of HFs are undergoing anagen at any given time, while the rest of the HFs are in the catagen or telogen phases (Trueb 2010). The length of anagen for scalp HFs is approximately 2-6 years, while HFs of other body sites have much shorter anagen (1-6 months) (Habif 2010). The onset of anagen and the resumption of mitotic activity in the hair bulb is dependent on an interaction between the dermal papilla and the overlying follicular epithelium (Paus & Cotsarelis 1999). In this phase, a new hair shaft begins to form at a rate of about 0.35 mm/day after the follicle grows down to meet the dermal papilla (Habif 2010). Since anagen hairs are rooted deeply in the dermis, they are more difficult to detach than hairs in other phases of the hair cycle (Cheng & Baylisss 2008). At the end of anagen, HFs enter the catagen phase, a 2-3 week transitional stage marked by widespread apoptosis of follicular keratinocytes as well as the degeneration and retraction of the outer root sheath around the lower bulb of the hair shaft (Habif 2010). The lower portion of the HF shrinks away from the underlying dermal papilla, which itself condenses and relocates to the level of the arrectorpili insertion point and bulge cells (Habif 2010). This relocation of the papilla to the bulge region of the HF is vital for the continuation of the hair cycle (Paus & Cotsarelis 1999). During the subsequent telogen, a phase of relative quiescence with no obvious structural changes, the hair shaft matures into a club hair and is eventually ejected by the growing follicle or physically removed by brushing or washing. This phase lasts for about 2-3 months until anagen commences again (Paus & Cotsarelis 1999; Habif 2010). Approximately 5-15% of the scalp HFs are in telogen at any given time (Paus & Cotsarelis 1999).

Clinical Features of Chemotherapy-Induced Alopecia

As previously discussed, during the anagen phase of the hair cycle, matrix cells undergo rapid proliferation to build the growing hair shaft. In response to chemotherapy treatment, the mitotic activity of these proliferating cells is abruptly terminated, leading to the weakening of the partially keratinized proximal portion of the hair shaft (Trueb 2010). The result is anagen effluvium, an increase in the breakage of anagen hairs and hair shedding.

For people who experience chemotherapy-induced alopecia, hair loss usually begins within 1-3 weeks of chemotherapy initiation, although it becomes most severe within 1-2 months (Batchelor 2001). Hair loss usually occurs in a patchy distribution, depending on how much of the hair is undergoing anagen at the time of treatment (Chon *et al.* 2012). Most patients experience hair regrowth at 3-6 months after the first dose of chemotherapy, and although sometimes the hair may show changes in color and/or texture, this is usually temporary (Munstedt *et al.* 1997). In rare cases, CIA may remain permanent (Miteva *et al.* 2011). The incidence and severity of CIA varies depending on the cytotoxic agent used, its route of administration, dose and dosing schedule, and the response of the individual (Chon *et al.* 2012). Differences in the incidence of CIA have been documented between major classes of chemotherapy drugs: 80% for antimicrotubule agents such as paclitaxel, 60-100% for topoisomerase inhibitors such as etoposide, 60% for alkylators such as cyclophosphamide, and 10-50% for antimetabolites (Trueb 2010).

It has also been shown that combination therapies produce a higher incidence and severity of alopecia than when single agents.(Trueb 2010).

Early Animal Models of Chemotherapy-Induced Alopecia

The lack of experimental animal models had relegated CIA as a purely observational disorder. However in a seminal paper published in Nature in 1969, Homan et al first made the observation that cyclophosphamide administered to poodles, angora rabbits and Suffolk sheep induced hair loss (Homan *et al.* 1969). In the Suffolk sheep, alopecia was observed only in actively proliferating HF on the trunk and not on the face, ears and limbs, since HFs in those areas were of a different type and grew in a different cycle (Homan *et al.* 1969). Cyclophosphamide was therefore proposed as a defleecing agent (Dolnick *et al.* 1969). Dolnick et al observed that after 7 days of cyclophosphamide administration, fleece could be easily removed without the need for shearing. Feil et al performed similar work in sheep and found that cyclophosphamide as well as Iphosphamide were effectively alopecic, while Trophosphamide was not (Feil & Lamoureux 1974). These findings indicated that chemotherapy was as deleterious to proliferating HFs in animals as it was in humans. While these models provided proof of principle of the alopecic effect of chemotherapy across species, they were expensive and difficult to work with, factors that significantly hampered the use of CIA models.

Development of the Rat and Mouse Models

There was a significant hiatus in the field of CIA animal research until the rat neonatal model was introduced in 1990 by a serendipitous observation (Hussein *et al.* 1990). While working with chemotherapy in young Sprague-Dawley rats and neonates, Hussein et al observed that young rats would lose their body hair completely at certain times. After much experimentation, it was observed that CIA ensued only during the anagen phase of the HF. In their first publication, the authors demonstrated that the use of chemotherapies that were alopecic to humans also resulted in the development of CIA in rat neonates (Hussein *et al.* 1990). For the first time, a reproducible and cost-efficient model for CIA was available to researchers worldwide (Hussein 1993).

Following the establishment of the young Sprague-Dawley rat model, an adult mouse model was developed for CIA (Paus *et al.* 1994). Synchronized anagen was induced by physical depilation (plucking) in adult C57BL/-6 mice that had undergone a complete postnatal hair cycle, so that the dorsal skin closely mimics the human scalp, where the vast majority of the HFs are in anagen (Paus *et al.* 1994). Additionally, a young mouse model was developed using conditions adapted from the previously established young rat model (Jimenez *et al.* 2008). Another neonatal rat model was also developed using Wistar rats instead of the Sprague-Dawley rats used initially, following similar principles as the first model (Nakashima-Kaminmura *et al.* 2008). Finally and more recently, Wikramanayake et al developed a pigmented, adult rat model for CIA using the Long-Evans rat strain (Wikramanayake *et al.* 2012a). Unlike in the adult mouse model where anagen was synchronized via plucking of the hairs, in this model hairs were clipped in early telogen to induce synchronized anagen. Thus, Wikramanayake et al established the first pigmented adult rat model for CIA, using the non-invasive and efficient means of hair clipping for synchronization.

In addition to these mouse and rat models in which chemotherapy agents were administered during one anagen phase, a multi-course rat model of CIA has been developed recently (Wikramanayake *et al.*)In this model, chemotherapy agents are given during the postnatal HF morphogenesis and subsequent, synchronized anagen stages. This model with multi-course treatment resembles the chemotherapy in patients more closely than single anagen models.

Together, these mouse and rat models provide invaluable tools not only to further our understanding of the cellular and molecular mechanisms underlying CIA, but also to evaluate novel therapeutics aimed at preventing or ameliorating CIA.

Furthermore, the multi-course model can be used to assess the effects of alopecia-preventing compounds during the first round of chemotherapy (such as chloroleukemia) and during subsequent rounds of chemotherapy in cancer survivors.

Histopathology of Chemotherapy-Induced Alopecia in Rodents

Hendrix et al carried out a comprehensive analysis of the morphological damage in HFs in response to chemotherapy using the mouse model of cyclophosphamide-induced CIA (Hendrix *et al.* 2005). Depending on the severity of the damage by the cytotoxic agent, the HFs undergo either the "dystrophic anagen pathway" induced by a lower dose of cyclophosphamide (120mg/kg body weight), or the "dystrophic catagen pathway" induced by a higher dose (150mg/kg body weight). Because of the wave pattern of anagen HFs in the mouse and rat, dystrophy and alopecia also occur in a wave pattern from head to tail (Hendrix *et al.* 2005).

Dystrophic anagen is characterized by shedding of the hair shaft followed by an incomplete "primary recovery", which generates a faulty new hair shaft. This process is then followed by a normal catagen-telogen phase. Thereafter, a "secondary recovery" occurs in which a normal hair shaft is generated. Dystrophic anagen is also characterized by the location and the size of ectopic melanin granules or clumps. During mid-dystrophic anagen, melanogenesis is reduced but still intact (Hendrix *et al.* 2005). However, late dystrophic anagen HFs display hair shaft fragments and a loss of the stripe banding pattern. Additionally, the presence of apoptotic bodies detected by the TUNEL assay can help determine whether a HF is in early, mid- or late dystrophic anagen. Another parameter that aids in the determination of each phase is the bulb size compared with the size of the dermal papillae (DP) as well as the shape of the DP, which can be stained for alkaline phosphatase. Lastly, the hair canal is slightly widened, and in late dystrophic anagen, filled with hair shaft fragments.

Dystrophic catagen is characterized by an immediate entry into a dystrophic catagen without a primary recovery, followed by a dramatically shortened and dystrophic telogen leading to a secondary recovery (Paus *et al.* 1994). Early dystrophic catagen HFs are characterized by a follicular distortion, with the DP condensed and ball-shaped, in contrast to the spindle-like or swollen appearance of healthy or dystrophic anagen HFs. Large ectopic melanin clumps are found in the IRS, ORS, and connective tissue sheath. The bulb is reduced in size with more apoptotic bodies, and the hair canal is widened and filled with fragmented hair shaft (Hendrix *et al.* 2005). During mid-dystrophic catagen, no club hair is formed, in contrast to healthy catagen. In late dystrophic catagen, the trailing connective tissue sheath is filled with large melanin clumps, and remnants of the hair shaft can be found in the widened hair canal (Hendrix *et al.* 2005).

In accordance with these findings, Selleri et al later demonstrated that doxorubicin induced apoptosis in the perifollicular connective tissue sheath, and to some degree in the matrix near the DP (Selleri *et al.* 2004). They proposed that the remodeling of the mesenchymal compartment is one of the main events that lead to alopecia. In addition, they observed that the epithelial cells in the ORS had undergone oncosis during HF regression. In this regard, Amoh et al showed that doxorubicin disrupted the blood vessel network of the HFs, thereby causing a decrease in the blood vessels supplying blood to the HFs (Amoh *et al.* 2007).

Thus, it is clear that the HF structure is greatly damaged upon chemotherapy, underscoring the importance of understanding the morphological changes of the HFs in response to different chemotherapies. Dystrophic anagen or catagen has a direct correlation with the regrowth of hair, which can be modulated with cyclosporine A, dexamethasone and FK 506 (Paus *et al.* 1994; Maurer *et al.* 1997).

Protection from Chemotherapy-Induced Alopecia by Cytokines and Growth Factors

The first paper describing protection of HFs from chemotherapy was published in 1990(Hussein *et al.* 1990). Hussein et al showed that treatment with ImuVert, a biological response modifier derived from *Serratiamarcescens*, protected against full body alopecia in the young rat model of CIA induced by cytosine arabinoside (cytarabine) or doxorubicin, but not cyclophosphamide. More importantly, they were able to test the protective effect on the development of leukemia using a similar model of rat chloroleukemia (Jimenez & Yunis 1987). Since ImuVert is a biological response modifier, its mechanism of action is most likely through the release of cytokines. Shortly after this report was published, ImuVert, in combination with N-acetylcysteine, was shown to protect against alopecia induced by cyclophosphamide, applied topically or injected parenterally. Protection from CIA was also observed using N-acetylcysteine alone. These findings were extended to the protection of CIA induced by a combination of cytarabine and cyclophosphamide (Jimenez *et al.* 1992a). Using the same rat model, it was then reported that interleukin-1 protected against doxorubicin and cytarabine-induced CIA (Jimenez *et al.* 1991; Jimenez *et al.* 1992b). In later work, Tsuruki et al confirmed these results in young rats treated with N-formyl-Met-Leu-Phe and MMK-1, an agonist of the formyl peptide receptor (Tsuruki *et al.* 2007)N-formyl-Met-Leu-Phe receptor binding resulted in protection from etoposide-induced alopecia. The authors suggested that the mechanism of action of both compounds was through the activation of NF-κB through the interleukin-1 pathway downstream of the formyl peptide receptor-like 1.

In a separate study, Jimenez et al demonstrated that epidermal growth factor and fibroblast-growth factor-1 protected against cytarabine-induced alopecia (Jimenez & Yunis 1992a). Subsequently, based on the premise that keratinocyte growth factor stimulated keratinocytes in rat embryos and neonates, Danilenko et al tested recombinant keratinocyte growth factor on the young rat model of CIA induced by cytarabine, and observed a 50% protection rate when administered 1 day prior to chemotherapy.(Danilenko *et al.* 1995)

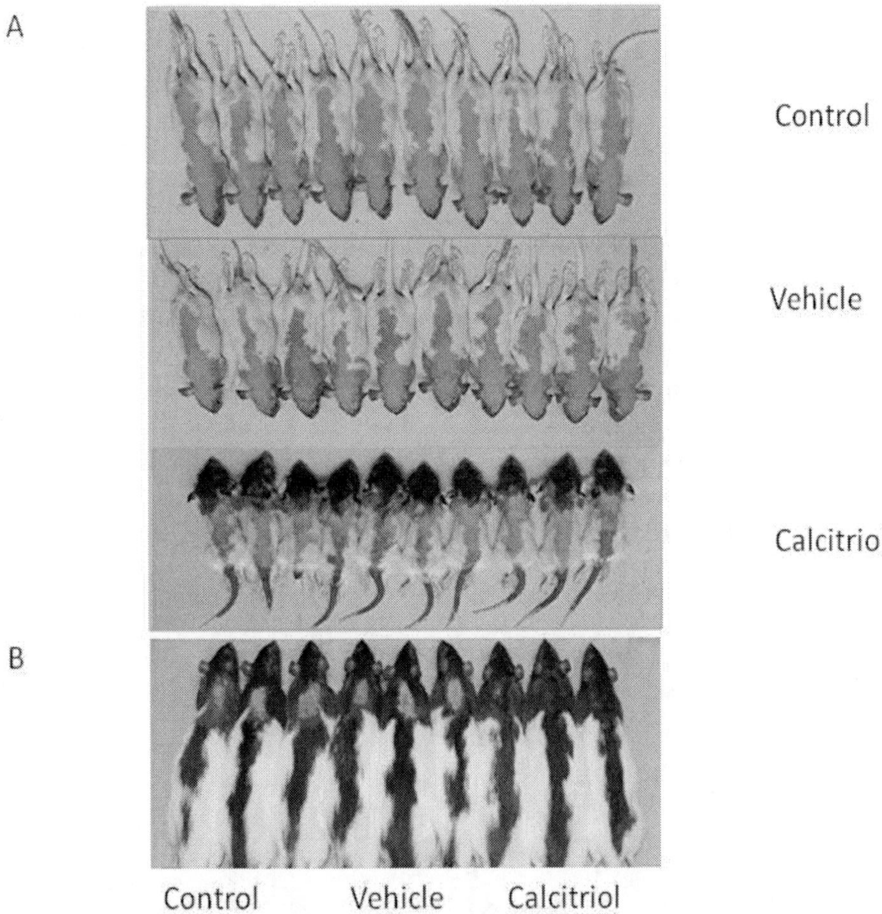

Figure 1. Prevention of chemotherapy-induced alopecia by Calcitriol in the multi-course rat model. (A) Chloroleukemia cells had been injected in Long-Evans rat pups on day 7 after birth. Cyclophosphamide was administered on day 11. Pups were then randomly divided into Control, Vehicle and Calcitriol groups and monitored for alopecia. Calcitriol (dissolved in ethanol) was applied topically on top of the head daily starting on day 6 and continued through day 11. The daily dose was 0.1µg in 0.1 ml of ethanol. Alopecia was recorded 10 days later.(B) Adult survivors of Shay's Chloroleukemia had hair clipping on the nape of the neck on day 21 after birth, and were treated with cyclophosphamide 15 days later. They were then randomized for Control, Vehicle and Calcitriol treatment, and monitored for alopecia. Vehicle (ethanol) and calcitriol were applied topically on the nape of the neck. The daily dose was 0.1µg in 0.1 ml of ethanol. Alopecia was recorded 10 days later. Notice that alopecia developed in the clipped areas in the control and vehicle-treated rats, but not in the Calcitriol-treated rats.

The immunomodulator AS101 has been demonstrated to exhibit chemoprotective effects in mice (Sredni *et al.* 1996). In a phase II clinical trial, 58 patients were treated either with AS101 and carboplatin/etoposide, or with chemotherapy alone. As observed in the murine model, a significant decrease in the level of alopecia was observed in patients receiving AS101. Using the rat model to investigate the underlying mechanism, the authors showed that protection by AS101, like ImuVert, may be mediated through the release of cytokines such as IL-1 (Sredni *et al.* 1996). Such studies provided proof-of-principle that the rodent models can serve as valid models of CIA, not only for therapeutic development, but also to investigate the underlying mechanisms of CIA.

Protection from Chemotherapy-Induced Alopecia by 1,25-dihydroxyvitamin D_3 (Calcitriol)

In 1992, Jimenez et al published a landmark paper that would lead to clinical trials aimed at solely treating CIA.(Jimenez & Yunis 1992b)In this study, the young rat model was used to test the chemoprotective properties of active metabolite of vitamin D3, 1,25-dihydroxy-vitamin D_3, also known as calcitriol. Their findings indicated that topical treatment with low doses of calcitriol protected against alopecia induced by etoposide, cyclophosphamide, doxorubicin and a combination of doxorubicin and cyclophosphamide (Jimenez & Yunis 1992b) (Figure 1 and 2). Calcitriol was also tested in the mouse model, and enhanced the hair regrowth post chemotherapy (Paus *et al.* 1996). It was suggested that calcitriol promoted a shift towards a state of dystrophic catagen, thereby entering the secondary recovery after an extremely shortened dystrophic telogen phase, which in turn translated to faster recovery rates.

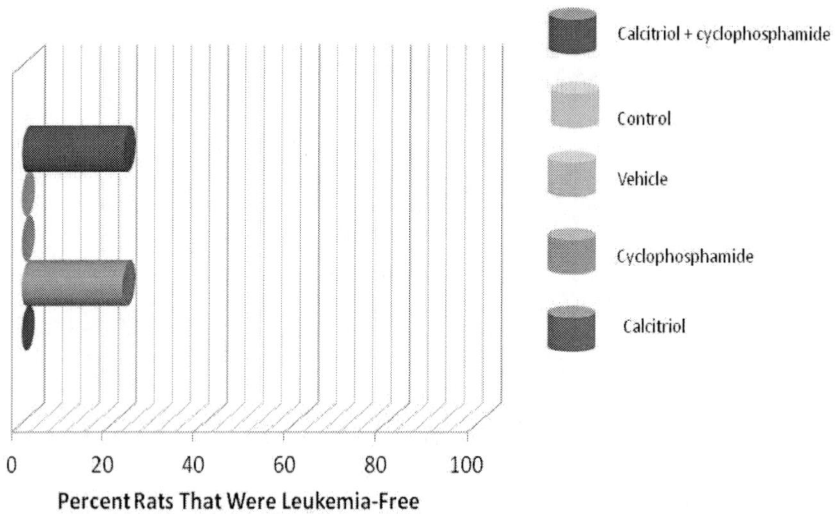

Figure 2. Topical calcitriol treatment did not diminish the effect of cyclophosphamide on Shay's Chloroleukemia, p= 0.8.

Chen et al, employed a modified version of the plucking mouse model by clipping instead of depilating to induce anagen (Chen *et al.* 1998). In their study, calcitriol protected male mice from CIA while females were only partially protected. However, this protective effect was attenuated in male mice but became more significant in female mice when they were inoculated with the EMT-6 murine mammary tumor prior to treatment. In fact, topical administration of calcitriol was additive in the effect of cyclophosphamide. In a later study, Schilli et al demonstrated that topical calcitriol pretreatment in mice significantly reduced HF matrix cell apoptosis induced by cyclophosphamide (Schilli *et al.* 1998). Interestingly, overexpression of Bcl-2, an apoptosis inhibitor, in the ORS keratinocytes under the control of the keratin-14 promoter, led to increased chemotherapy-associated keratinocyte apoptosis, HF dystrophy and alopecia (Muller-Rover *et al.* 1999; Muller-Rover *et al.* 2000).

Protection from Chemotherapy-Induced Alopecia by Hormones

In an independent study, it was hypothesized that parathyroid hormone, parathyroid related peptide and the parathyroid/parathyroid related peptide receptor, which are ubiquitously expressed in cutaneous tissue, may affect CIA (Peters *et al.* 2001). The authors demonstrated that parathyroid/parathyroid related peptide agonists ameliorated the effect of cyclophosphamide in a mouse model by shifting HFs to a state of dystrophic anagen, with decreased numbers of TUNEL-positive apoptotic cells, leading to a delay in cyclophosphamide-induced CIA. In sharp contrast, treatment with parathyroid hormone led to apoptosis with a dystrophic catagen phenotype, with increased alopecia but accelerated hair regrowth. In a later study, Katikaneni et al demonstrated that PTH agonists fused to the collagen binding domain (CBD) of *Clostridium histolyticum* resulted in more rapid hair regrowth and repigmentation, while no difference from chemotherapy alone was observed in the PTH-CBD antagonist group (Katikaneni *et al.* 2012). The linking of CBD to the PTH agonists and antagonists in this experiment facilitated the delivery and retention of the hormone to the skin. Similarly, Ohnemus et al showed that topical 17-β-estradiol, but not the estrogen antagonist ICI 182.780, altered the effect of HFs to chemotherapy by inducing the dystrophic catagen pathway which led to a decrease in hair regrowth time (Ohnemus *et al.* 2006). Control or ICI 182.780, on the other hand, exhibited dystrophic anagen leading to protracted hair regrowth.

Protection from Chemotherapy-Induced Alopecia by Inhibition of Apoptosis

Nakashima-Kamimuraet al demonstrated that the anti-apoptotic protein FNK protected against etoposide-induced alopecia in a rat model in a dose-dependent manner (Nakashima-Kaminmura *et al.* 2008). Furthermore, a human version of FNK also exhibited protective activity. These results indicate that FNK may provide an alternative to treat CIA. In this regard, M50054, an inhibitor of apoptosis, was found to protect mice from chemotherapy CIA when applied topically by way of inhibiting caspase 3 activation.(Tsuda *et al.* 2001) Botchkarev et al have demonstrated that CIA is dependent on the tumor suppressor p53(Botchkarev *et al.* 2000).p53 mouse mutants which exhibited Fas downregulation and insulin growth factor-binding 3 as well as bcl-2 upregulation were protected against CIA. Similarly, it was demonstrated that p53 target gene EDA2R is upregulated concomitantly with p53 during CIA (Brosh *et al.* 2010). However, it is not indispensable for the induction of CIA. The authors speculate that other targets for p53 may be required. Indeed Fas was reported to be elevated during CIA, but its abrogation did not confer protection from chemotherapy (Jimenez *et al.* 1991). Interestingly, lack of p53 did not prevent CIA in males, while it did in females, thereby indicating the activation of alternative mechanisms.(Brosh *et al.*)

Protection from Chemotherapy-Induced Alopecia by Activation of the Stress Response Mechanism

In 2008, a report using both the rat and mouse models demonstrated that induction of heat shock proteins by the administration of heat protected the HFs at the site of localized heat application from CIA (Jimenez *et al.* 2008). Follicles expressing heat shock protein 70 (HSPA1A) were protected from doxorubicin-, cyclophosphamide- and paclitaxel-induced dystrophy. Additionally, it was shown that administration of geldanamycin, an inducer of heat shock proteins, resulted in the localized protection from chemotherapy. Furthermore, it was demonstrated that heat shock induction had no effect on the development of induced leukemia or chemotherapy efficacy in the rat model. Thus, the activation of the stress mechanism was shown to confer protection of the HFs from chemotherapy toxicity.

Protection from Chemotherapy-Induced Alopecia by Sulfur-Containing Compounds

α-Lipoic acid is an anti-oxidant that has been shown to have beneficial effects in many areas of health. In a recent study, Hagiwara et al tested the effects of the α-Lipoic acid derivative, sodium zinc dihydrolipoylhistidinate (DHLHZn), in a young rat CIA model (Hagiwara *et al.* 2011). Rats treated with DHLHZn and AraC chemotherapy experienced significantly reduced CIA and inflammatory cell infiltration of the HFs than those treated with AraC alone. The anti-oxidant and anti-inflammatory effects of the DHLHZn may partly explain the mechanism behind the CIA attenuation observed. In a later study, D'Agostini et al demonstrated the effect of an oral administration of L-cystine and vitamin B6 in a young mouse model of CIA (D'Agostini *et al.* 2012). The sulfur-containing amino acid cysteine and its covalently linked dimer cystine are vital components of normal HF production, and Vitamin B6 is an essential cofactor involved in skin development and maintenance. Higher doses of L-cystine and vitamin B6 indeed prevented a significant decrease in hair in doxorubicin treated mice.

However, before extrapolating these results to the human, more research must be done to determine whether or not these treatments interfere with the anti-tumoral activity of chemotherapy.

Modulation of Hair Regrowth after Chemotherapy-Induced Alopecia

In separate studies conducted by Sato et al, it was demonstrated that overexpression of the sonic hedgehog gene, which is involved in the initiation of the hair cycle, did not protect against CIA, but led to increased post-chemothrapy regrowth (Sato *et al.* 2001).

In a study conducted by Selleri et al, the expression of caveolin-1 (a protein involved in cell proliferation and chemoresistance) and β-catenin was analyzed at different intervals pre- and post-doxorubicin administration in a mouse model (Selleri *et al.* 2005). Cells of the bulge area were positive for caveolin-1 during all phases of the hair cycle: anagen, catagen and telogen. β-catenin, on the other hand, was detected in the deeper portion of the HF but not in the bulge cells during anagen. Doxorubicin-treated HFs still expressed caveolin-1 in the bulge area; however β-catenin was negative throughout the HF. Thus, expression of caveolin-1 may confer protection to follicular progenitor cells. Abnormal melanogenesis was observed in mice treated with doxorubicin, in accordance to previous studies; however bulge stem cells were not involved.

Plonka et al demonstrated that oral $zinc^{2+}$ can delay but not protect against cyclophosphamide-induced alopecia (Plonka *et al.* 2005). Treatment with zinc post chemotherapy revealed that zinc given immediately after the onset of alopecia can aid in HF recovery; however, if administered later, it resulted in hair growth retardation.

Imanishi et al have studied the effect of laminin-511 and laminin-332 in CIA (Imanishi *et al.* 2010). Their observations indicate that laminin-332 and its receptor α6β4 integrin are upregulated after mid- to late dystrophic catagen induced by cyclophosphamide administration in mice. Conversely, laminin-511 is downregulated at the plateau of dystrophic catagen, although it can induce the α3 integrin system. However, when a laminin-511 extract but not recombinant laminin-332 was administered, it was observed that cyclophosphamide-dependent alopecia was delayed. These results indicate that laminin-511 can retard CIA and may induce hair regrowth, while laminin-332 is present in non-proliferative states.

Additionally, in a more recent study, Wikramanayake et al used the young rat model to test the effect of low-level laser treatment on hair regrowth after CIA (Wikramanayake *et al.* 2012c). Low-energy photobiomodulation has been used in medicine since the 1960s, and is increasingly becoming more widely used in many medical situations due to its positive safety profile (Metelitsa & Green ; Brosseau *et al.* 2000; Bjordal *et al.* 2003; Hawkins *et al.* 2005; Schubert *et al.* 2007). The HairMaxLaserComb® has been approved by the FDA for the treatment of androgenetic alopecia (Leavitt *et al.* 2009), and a modified device was recently shown to induce hair regrowth in a mouse model for alopecia areata (Wikramanayake *et al.* 2012b). In this study, the authors showed that the laser treatment significantly reduced the time for hair regrowth, but did not affect the efficacy of chemotherapy. Thus, low-level laser treatment should be explored as a safe and user-friendly option to modulate CIA in patients.

Animal Models and Clinical Trials

The seminal discovery of the chemoprotective effects of 1,25-dihydroxyvitamin D_3 on CIA (Jimenez & Yunis 1992b) led to two phase-I clinical trials, but neither showed significant protection against CIA (Hidalgo *et al.* 1999; Bleiker *et al.* 2005) In one study, the lack of efficacy may be partly due to poor scalp penetration of calcitriol using a cream formulation (Hidalgo *et al.* 1999). In the other study, a scalp solution of calcipotriol was used and penetrability was not tested (Bleiker *et al.* 2005). In addition, pretreatment was carried out for only four days, not taking into account that the hair cycles in humans are much more prolonged when compared with rodents. Furthermore, dosing and treatment regimen may not have been optimal. Indeed, when calcitriol was administered one day prior to chemotherapy, or on the same day of chemotherapy in the young rat model, no protection was observed (unpublished results). Thus, extrapolation of the use of 1,25-dihydroxyvitamin D3 in human trials will require extensive optimization of formulation, dose, frequency and duration.

Conclusion

Animal models, murine models in particular, have shed important light into the pathogenesis of CIA. They have highlighted the cytotoxic damage to HF matrix cells during chemotherapy. More importantly, they allow in-depth dissection of the mediators and pathways involved. A better insight into the underlying mechanisms will ultimately lead to an array of therapeutic interventions, which can be tested in these models prior to clinical trials. Effective amelioration and prevention of CIA will significantly improve the quality of life for cancer patients undergoing or considering chemotherapy, and may help improve compliance and efficacy of cancer treatment.

References

Amoh Y, Li L, Katsuoka K, Hoffman RM (2007). Chemotherapy targets the hair-follicle vascular network but not the stem cells. *J Invest Dermatol*. 127, 11-15.

Batchelor D (2001). Hair and cancer chemotherapy: consequences and nursing care--a literature study. *Eur J Cancer Care (Engl)*. 10, 147-163.

Bjordal JM, Couppe C, Chow RT, Tuner J, Ljunggren EA (2003). A systematic review of low level laser therapy with location-specific doses for pain from chronic joint disorders. *Aust J Physiother*. 49, 107-116.

Bleiker TO, Nicolaou N, Traulsen J, Hutchinson PE (2005). 'Atrophic telogen effluvium' from cytotoxic drugs and a randomized controlled trial to investigate the possible protective effect of pretreatment with a topical vitamin D analogue in humans. *Br J Dermatol*. 153, 103-112.

Botchkarev VA, Komarova EA, Siebenhaar F, Botchkareva NV, Komarov PG, Maurer M, Gilchrest BA, Gudkov AV (2000). p53 is essential for chemotherapy-induced hair loss. *Cancer Res*. 60, 5002-5006.

Brosh R, Sarig R, Natan EB, Molchadsky A, Madar S, Bornstein C, Buganim Y, Shapira T, Goldfinger N, Paus R, Rotter V p53-dependent transcriptional regulation of EDA2R and its involvement in chemotherapy-induced hair loss. *FEBS Lett.* 584, 2473-2477.

Brosh R, Sarig R, Natan EB, Molchadsky A, Madar S, Bornstein C, Buganim Y, Shapira T, Goldfinger N, Paus R, Rotter V (2010). p53-dependent transcriptional regulation of EDA2R and its involvement in chemotherapy-induced hair loss. *FEBS Lett.* 584, 2473-2477.

Brosseau L, Welch V, Wells G, deBie R, Gam A, Harman K, Morin M, Shea B, Tugwell P (2000). Low level laser therapy (classes I, II and III) in the treatment of rheumatoid arthritis. *Cochrane Database Syst Rev*, CD002049.

Chen G, Baechle A, Nevins TD, Oh S, Harmon C, Stacey DW (1998). Protection against cyclophosphamide-induced alopecia and inhibition of mammary tumor growth by topical 1,25-dihydroxyvitamin D3 in mice. *Int J Cancer.* 75, 303-309.

Cheng A, Baylisss S (2008). The Genetics of Hair Shaft Disorders. *J Am Acad Dermatol.* 59, 1-22.

Chon S, Champion R, Geddes E, Rashid R (2012). Chemotherapy-induced alopecia. *J Am Acad Dermatol.* 67, e37-47.

D'Agostini F, Fiallo P, Ghio M, Flora S (2012). Chemoprevention of doxorubicin-induced alopecia in mice by dietary administration of L-cystine and vitamin B6. *Arch Dermatol Res.* Ahead of print.

Danilenko DM, Ring BD, Yanagihara D, Benson W, Wiemann B, Starnes CO, Pierce GF (1995). Keratinocyte growth factor is an important endogenous mediator of hair follicle growth, development, and differentiation. Normalization of the nu/nu follicular differentiation defect and amelioration of chemotherapy-induced alopecia. *Am J Pathol.* 147, 145-154.

Dolnick EH, Lindahl IL, Terrill CE, Reynolds PJ (1969). Cyclophosphamide as a chemical "defleecing" agent for sheep. *Nature.* 221, 467-468.

Feil VJ, Lamoureux CH (1974). Alopecia activity of cyclophosphamide metabolites and related compounds in sheep. *Cancer Res.* 34, 2596-2598.

Habif T (2010). *Clinical Dermatology, 5th ed.*: Elsevier.

Hagiwara S, Uchida T, Koga H, Inomata M, Yoshizumi F, Moriyama M, Kitano S, Noguchi T (2011). The a-Lipoic Acid Derivative Sodium Zinc Dihydrolipoylhistidinate Reduces Chemotherapy-Induced Alopecia in a Rat Model: A Pilot Study. *Surg Today.* 41, 693-697.

Hawkins D, Houreld N, Abrahamse H (2005). Low level laser therapy (LLLT) as an effective therapeutic modality for delayed wound healing. *Ann N Y Acad Sci.* 1056, 486-493.

Hendrix S, Handjiski B, Peters EM, Paus R (2005). A guide to assessing damage response pathways of the hair follicle: lessons from cyclophosphamide-induced alopecia in mice. *J Invest Dermatol.* 125, 42-51.

Hidalgo M, Rinaldi D, Medina G, Griffin T, Turner J, Von Hoff DD (1999). A phase I trial of topical topitriol (calcitriol, 1,25-dihydroxyvitamin D3) to prevent chemotherapy-induced alopecia. *Anticancer Drugs.* 10, 393-395.

Homan ER, Zendzian RP, Busey WM, Rall DP (1969). Loss of hair in experimental animals induced by cyclophosphamide. *Nature.* 221, 1058-1059.

Hussein AM (1993). Chemotherapy-induced alopecia: new developments. *South Med J.* 86, 489-496.

Hussein AM, Jimenez JJ, McCall CA, Yunis AA (1990). Protection from chemotherapy-induced alopecia in a rat model. *Science*. 249, 1564-1566.

Imanishi H, Tsuruta D, Tateishi C, Sugawara K, Paus R, Tsuji T, Ishii M, Ikeda K, Kunimoto H, Nakajima K, Jones JC, Kobayashi H (2010). Laminin-511, inducer of hair growth, is down-regulated and its suppressor in hair growth, laminin-332 up-regulated in chemotherapy-induced alopecia. *J Dermatol Sci*. 58, 43-54.

Jimenez J, Huang HS, Yunis AA (1992a). Treatment with ImuVert/N-acetylcysteine protects rats from cyclophosphamide/cytarabine-induced alopecia. *Cancer Invest*. 10, 271-276.

Jimenez J, Sawaya ME, Yunis AA (1992b). Interleukin 1 protects hair follicles from cytarabine (ARA-C)-induced toxicity in vivo and in vitro. *FASEB J*. 6, 911-913.

Jimenez J, Wong GH, Yunis AA (1991). Interleukin 1 protects from cytosine arabinosdie-induced alopecia in the rat model. *FASEB J*. 5, 2456-2458.

Jimenez J, Yunis AA (1987). Tumor cell rejection through terminal cell differentiation. *Science*. 238, 1278-1280.

Jimenez J, Yunis AA (1992a). Protection from 1-beta-D-arabinofuranosylcytosine-induced alopecia by epidermal growth factor and fibroblast growth factor in the rat model. *Cancer Res*. 52, 413-415.

Jimenez JJ, Roberts SM, Mejia J, Mauro LM, Munson JW, Elgart GW, Connelly EA, Chen Q, Zou J, Goldenberg C, Voellmy R (2008). Prevention of chemotherapy-induced alopecia in rodent models. *Cell Stress Chaperones*. 13, 31-38.

Jimenez JJ, Yunis AA (1992b). Protection from chemotherapy-induced alopecia by 1,25-dihydroxyvitamin D3. *Cancer Res*. 52, 5123-5125.

Katikaneni R, Ponnapakkam T, Suda H, Miyata S, Sakon J, Matsushita O, Gensure R (2012). Treatment for chemotherapy-induced alopecia in mice using parathyroid hormone agonists and antagonists linked to a collagen binding domain. *Int J Cancer*. 131, E813-E821.

Leavitt M, Charles G, Heyman E, Michaels D (2009). HairMax LaserComb laser phototherapy device in the treatment of male androgenetic alopecia: A randomized, double-blind, sham device-controlled, multicentre trial. *Clin Drug Investig*. 29, 283-292.

Maurer M, Handjiski B, Paus R (1997). Hair growth modulation by topical immunophilin ligands: induction of anagen, inhibition of massive catagen development, and relative protection from chemotherapy-induced alopecia. *Am J Pathol*. 150, 1433-1441.

McGarvey EL, Baum LD, Pinkerton RC, Rogers LM (2001). Psychological sequelae and alopecia among women with cancer. *Cancer Practice*. 9, 283-289.

Metelitsa AI, Green JB Home-use laser and light devices for the skin: an update. *Semin Cutan Med Surg*. 30, 144-147.

Miteva M, Misciali C, Fanti PA, Vincenzi C, Romanelli P, Tosti A (2011). Permanent alopecia after systemic chemotherapy: a clinicopathological study of 10 cases. *Am J Dermatopathol*. 33, 345-350.

Muller-Rover S, Rossiter H, Lindner G, Peters EM, Kupper TS, Paus R (1999). Hair follicle apoptosis and Bcl-2. *J Investig Dermatol Symp Proc*. 4, 272-277.

Muller-Rover S, Rossiter H, Paus R, Handjiski B, Peters EM, Murphy JE, Mecklenburg L, Kupper TS (2000). Overexpression of Bcl-2 protects from ultraviolet B-induced apoptosis but promotes hair follicle regression and chemotherapy-induced alopecia. *Am J Pathol*. 156, 1395-1405.

Munstedt K, Manthey N, Sachsse S, Vahrson H (1997). Changes in self-concept and body image during alopecia induced cancer chemotherapy. *Support Care Cancer*. 5, 139-143.

Nakashima-Kaminmura N, Nishimaki K, Mori T, Asoh S, Ohta S (2008). Prevention of chemotherapy-induced alopecia by the anti-death FNK protein. *Life Sciences*. 82, 218.

Ohnemus U, Uenalan M, Inzunza J, Gustafsson JA, Paus R (2006). The hair follicle as an estrogen target and source. *Endocr Rev*. 27, 677-706.

Paus R, Cotsarelis G (1999). The Biology of Hair Follicles. *N Engl J Med*. 341, 491-497.

Paus R, Handjiski B, Eichmuller S, Czarnetzki BM (1994). Chemotherapy-induced alopecia in mice. Induction by cyclophosphamide, inhibition by cyclosporine A, and modulation by dexamethasone. *Am J Pathol*. 144, 719-734.

Paus R, Schilli MB, Handjiski B, Menrad A, Henz BM, Plonka P (1996). Topical calcitriol enhances normal hair regrowth but does not prevent chemotherapy-induced alopecia in mice. *Cancer Res*. 56, 4438-4443.

Peters EM, Foitzik K, Paus R, Ray S, Holick MF (2001). A new strategy for modulating chemotherapy-induced alopecia, using PTH/PTHrP receptor agonist and antagonist. *J Invest Dermatol*. 117, 173-178.

Plonka PM, Handjiski B, Popik M, Michalczyk D, Paus R (2005). Zinc as an ambivalent but potent modulator of murine hair growth in vivo- preliminary observations. *Exp Dermatol*. 14, 844-853.

Sato N, Leopold PL, Crystal RG (2001). Effect of adenovirus-mediated expression of Sonic hedgehog gene on hair regrowth in mice with chemotherapy-induced alopecia. *J Natl Cancer Inst*. 93, 1858-1864.

Schilli MB, Paus R, Menrad A (1998). Reduction of intrafollicular apoptosis in chemotherapy-induced alopecia by topical calcitriol-analogs. *J Invest Dermatol*. 111, 598-604.

Schubert MM, Eduardo FP, Guthrie KA, Franquin JC, Bensadoun RJ, Migliorati CA, Lloid CM, Eduardo CP, Walter NF, Marques MM, Hamdi M (2007). A phase III randomized double-blind placebo-controlled clinical trial to determine the efficacy of low level laser therapy for the prevention of oral mucositis in patients undergoing hematopoietic cell transplantation. *Support Care Cancer*. 15, 1145-1154.

Selleri S, Arnaboldi F, Palazzo M, Hussein U, Balsari A, Rumio C (2005). Caveolin-1 is expressed on multipotent cells of hair follicles and might be involved in their resistance to chemotherapy. *Br J Dermatol*. 153, 506-513.

Selleri S, Arnaboldi F, Vizzotto L, Balsari A, Rumio C (2004). Epithelium-mesenchyme compartment interaction and oncosis on chemotherapy-induced hair damage. *Lab Invest*. 84, 1404-1417.

Shimomura Y, Christiano AM (2010). Biology and genetics of hair. *Annu Rev Genomics Hum Genet*. 11, 109-132.

Sredni B, Xu RH, Albeck M, Gafter U, Gal R, Shani A, Tichler T, Shapira J, Bruderman I, Catane R, Kaufman B, Whisnant JK, Mettinger KL, Kalechman Y (1996). The protective role of the immunomodulator AS101 against chemotherapy-induced alopecia studies on human and animal models. *Int J Cancer*. 65, 97-103.

Trueb RM (2010). Chemotherapy-induced alopecia. *Current Opinion on Supportive and Palliative Care*. 4, 281-284.

Tsuda T, Ohmori Y, Muramatsu H, Hosaka Y, Takiguchi K, Saitoh F, Kato K, Nakayama K, Nakamura N, Nagata S, Mochizuki H (2001). Inhibitory effect of M50054, a novel inhibitor of apoptosis, on anti-Fas-antibody-induced hepatitis and chemotherapy-induced alopecia. *Eur J Pharmacol.* 433, 37-45.

Tsuruki T, Takahata K, Yoshikawa M (2007). Mechanism of the protective effect of intraperitoneally administered agonists for formyl peptide receptors against chemotherapy-induced alopecia. *Biosci Biotechnol Biochem.* 71, 1198-1202.

Wikramanayake TC, Amini S, Simon J, Mauro L, Elgart GW, Schachner L, Jimenez J (2012a). A novel rat model for chemotherapy-induced alopecia. *Clin Exp Dermatol.* 37, 284-289.

Wikramanayake TC, Amini S, Simon J, Mauro LM, Elgart G, Schachner LA, Jimenez JJ A novel rat model for chemotherapy-induced alopecia. *Clin Exp Dermatol.* 37, 284-289.

Wikramanayake TC, Rodriguez R, Choudhary S, Mauro LM, Nouri K, Schachner LA, Jimenez J (2012b). Effects of the Lexington LaserComb on hair regrowth in the C3H/HeJ mouse model of alopecia areata. *Lasers Med Sci.* 27, 431-436.

Wikramanayake TC, Villasante A, Mauro L, Nouri K, Schachner L, Perez C, Jimenez J (2012c). Low-level laser treatment accelerated hair regrowth in a rat model of chemotherapy-induced alopecia (CIA). *Lasers in Medical Science.* Ahead of Print.

In: Animal Models in Cancer Research …
Editor: Sean A. Murray

ISBN: 978-1-62417-587-9

Chapter VI

Murine Models of Human Colorectal Cancer: Techniques and Limitations

Jasneet Singh Bhullar [*] ***and Vijay K. Mittal***
Department of Surgery, Providence Hospital and Medical Centers,
Southfield, Michigan, US

Abstract

Murine models of colon carcinogenesis are an essential tool in understanding the mechanisms of pathogenesis and to evaluate therapeutic and preventive measures. Over the years considerable changes in the understanding of the murine models of human colon cancer has resulted in numerous models being reported in the literature. The reports of colon cancer transgenic mice were followed by human xenograft heterotopic murine models. With the orthotopic tumor models being found to be more relevant in portraying the human disease process as opposed to heterotopic models, many techniques for making orthotopic colorectal murine models were reported. Although all of these models have their advantages and limitations, the latest orthotopic murine models seem to accurately represent and replicate the human disease process.

We discuss the different human colon cancer murine models, their background, the technique of creating them along with their advantages and limitations. This extensive overview and details of an array of different resources in this field offers the researchers a wide choice to choose a model which is more applicable to the type of study being planned.

Keywords: Animals; anticarcinogenic Agents; therapeutic use; diagnostic use; chemoprevention; colonic neoplasms; chemically induced; prevention and control; diet disease models; mice; mouse; murine; mutant strains; precancerous conditions; animal model; diet; chemoprevention; colon-carcinogenesis; min-mice; colon cancer; colorectal cancer; xenograft; heterotopic model; orthotopic model; murine model

[*] Address for correspondence, Jasneet Singh Bhullar MD, MS, Department of Surgery, Providence Hospital & Medical Centers, 16001 West 9 Mile Road, Southfield, MI 48075, USA, Phone: 248-849-7638, Fax: 248-849-5380, Email: drjsbhullar@gmail.com.

Introduction

Colorectal carcinoma (CRC)is the second most common cause of cancer mortality among men as well as women in the United States. Much research is being done to study the pathogenesis, epidemiological factors, potential chemoprevention and therapeutic options. The molecular genetic studies have identified several key genes whose mutations or altered expression can cause CRC. Also, recent years have seen an explosion in the molecular understanding of CRC, which has led to the development of not only more effective cytotoxic cancer drugs but also more potentially cytostatic or ant metastatic agents as well.

Useful animal models of colorectal carcinogenesis are needed not only to study the mechanisms of pathogenesis, but also to investigate potential therapeutic and preventive measures and are an essential part of the ongoing oncology research. The laboratory mouse (*Muss muscles*) has become one of the best animal model species in biomedical research today because of: 1) The availability of genetic/genomic information 2) Precise and well-established mutagenesis techniques to construct transgenic and knockout mice and 3) Chemical mutagenesis technologies [1].

Rodents and humans share many biological functions, and rodents are invaluable for toxicity tests. Rodent studies are also needed in the chemoprevention area, because epidemiological studies do not lead to firm conclusions as confounding factors cannot be fully eliminated. Thus, the hypotheses generated by epidemiology must be tested in controlled experiments, ideally in a human population [2]. However this is a very long and costly process, with moral and ethical complications, and it could jeopardize the health of the volunteers. Thus, animal trials should precede human trials of innovations in treatment and prevention of colorectal carcinoma.

Both basic science studies and clinical trials are essential components of the cancer drug discovery process. Trial drugs found to be significantly better than no treatment or standard therapies (*i.e.,* active) in preclinical laboratory cancer models or compounds with novel chemo types and equivalent effectiveness to standard treatments are advanced to confirmatory testing in early (Phase I and II) clinical trials. A favorable response rate in Phase II trials advances a drug into additional clinical testing and is considered a prerequisite of drug success in the clinic setting [3].

Advancement of a trial drug from preclinical testing in the laboratory to testing in Phase II clinical trials is based on the assumption that drug activity in cancer models translates into at least some efficacy in human patients, *i.e.,* that cancer laboratory models are clinically predictive.

Major differences between rodents and humans in lifespan, body weight, intestinal morphology (e.g. cecum), gut micro flora, way of eating and digestion (e.g. meals, chewing, coprophagia), and gene regulation may change the outcome of dietary interventions.

The use of preclinical cancer models for selection of potential cancer therapeutics was pioneered by the National Cancer Institute (NCI) in the United States in the mid-1950s. Subsequently, in 1990, the NCI introduced a disease-oriented *in vitro* Human Tumor Cell Line Screen comprised of 60 cell lines from the most common adult tumors [4-6]. The screen was designed so that each tumor type was represented by a panel of cell lines, selected on the basis of different subhistological features, and common drug resistance profiles. It was hoped that this screen would help identify drug leads with high potency and/or selective activity against particular tumor types.

The NCI had examined the correlation between drug activity in Phase II clinical trials and preclinical activity in cancer models [7], which showed that with the exception of breast and colon histologies, human xenografts did not significantly predict Phase II clinical activity in other cancers types. The results from multiple studies [3,8,9,10] have shown that *in vitro* cell lines (in the context of the NCI Human Tumor Cell Line Screen) and appropriate panels of the human xenograft model have significant advantages over the murine allograft model in drug development. Over the years more than 100,000 rodents have been sacrificed in the quest for chemoprevention. It was concluded that rodent studies are extremely useful to screen for potential chemopreventive agents and to eliminate agents that have no effect or promote tumor growth (this number was estimated from the colon cancer chemoprevention database, http://corpet.net/min, and includes liver, mammary, esophagus, pancreas, prostate, and skin cancer studies). It may therefore be prudent to use rodent models as screening tools; agents which turn out to be ineffective or tumor-promoting in rodents should not be tested in a human population [11]. An appropriate role for animals in cancer chemoprevention is thus the ''initial screen''. Such screens may well discover as yet unknown potent chemopreventive agents [2]. Murine cancer models can also allow the study of mechanisms to help identify new biomarkers and novel target genes. Mechanisms can be studied because invasive procedures and the use of toxic compounds pose less ethical problems in rodents than in humans. Moreover, less time and money are required to test a hypothesis in rodents than in humans [11]. Once biomarkers and novel genes are identified in mice, they can subsequently be detected in humans. Novel gene targets were identified in human tumors on the basis of evidence collected from transcriptional profiles in Min mice [12]. Keeping in mind all of the extensive studies on murine cancer models, it is obvious that human beings will not be able to find new ways to prevent cancer without the help of animal models. This is especially true in the case of CRC. The challenge of murine models of CRC is that rodents have almost no spontaneous CRC, therefore a carcinogen is needed to induce the tumors [11]. Transgenic mouse strains that spontaneously develop CRC closely imitate human cancer syndromes, such as hereditary nonpolyposis colorectal cancer (HNPCC) [13] and familial adenomatosis polyposis (FAP) [14]. These models have proven to be invaluable for the study of the effects of known genetic alterations on the disease course. However, many of these mouse models form adenomas primarily in the small intestine, and are typically associated with a slow growth rate and considerable inter-animal variability [1]. Thus the human CRC murine model remains the essential tool for research on human CRC.

Colorectal Cancer Cell Lines

With increasing basic and translational research on CRC worldwide, the demand for commercially available CRC cell lines has been on the rise. In keeping up with this demand, more than one hundred different CRC cell lines of human as well as murine origin are available from the American Type Culture Collection (ATCC, Manassas, VA; www.atcc.org) and the NCI Frederick Laboratory for Cancer Research (Frederick, MD). These cell lines have a well documented origin, characteristics, morphology and DNA profile. They have been extensively characterized in various in vitro and in vivo systems, including invasive and metastatic properties, genetic aberrations, drug response and expression of cancer - associated genes [15]. Having the details of such an array of different cell lines offers the researchers a wide choice of a pertinent cell lines which are more applicable to the type of study being planned. Because of the accumulated knowledge, these well-described cell lines are attractive for use in tumor models, provided that cell lines relevant for the purpose of the study are selected.

Flatmark *et al.* evaluated the commonly available human CRC cell lines in an orthotopic model to determine which lines would be best suited to investigate the process of spontaneous metastasis. The results showed considerable differences between the cell lines with respect to 'take' rate, growth rate and metastatic ability, resulting in a panel of tumors that seem to reflect a heterogeneity that may be clinically relevant [15]. The twelve CRC lines evaluated were Co205, HCT15, HCT116, Colo320DM, SW480, SW620, CaCo2, HT29, WiDr, KM20L2, HCC2998 and Co115. Six of the 12 cell lines had 'take' rates of 100%(KM20L2, HCT116, HCT15, SW480, SW620 and Colo320DM), whereas intermediate ‘take’ rates were observed for Co115 (90%), HCC2998 (88%) and HT29(69%). The lymph-node metastases were noted with the highest frequencies for HCC2998 and HT29 cell line groups.

Kuo and colleagues [16] had previously studied eight CRC cell lines (including Co205 and WiDr) in a similar orthotopic model, in which subcutaneous xenografts were sutured to the cecum following scraping of the serosa surface. They had reported high ‘take’ rates (100%) for all cell lines tested, while in the study done by Flatmak *et al.* the ‘take’ rates for theCo205 and WiDr were rather low (40%) [15]. There was no obvious explanation for these observed differences, but they might be attributed to the common experience that cell lines may differ in characteristics when studied indifferent laboratories. Also, the differences in results obtained in vivo with the same cell lines in different institutions might also be related to the use of different strains of mice. It is still unclear, however, to what influence the genetic composition of immunodeficient mice has for a consistent and convincing effect on the 'take' rate and growth of human tumors [17].

Depending on which cell line is selected by the researcher for the study, the cells are cultivated under recommended conditions, and they are usually detached with trypsin–EDTA. After counting the tumor cells, the usual injection number is $1X10^6$ cells/mouse.

Xenograft Murine Colorectal Cancer Models

Immunodeficient mice are used to establish a xenograft murine model. Depending upon the researcher's choice, either BALB/c nude (nu/nu) mice or NOD *SCID* mice are preferred. Sometimes females are used more often than males for the convenience of housing the animals, as female mice can be housed together in a single cage while males usually need to housed individually.

1. Heterotopic Models

The subcutaneous xenograft heterotopic model is made by injectionof1X10^{6} tumor cells/site within the subcutaneous tissues of flank/hind leg of the mouse. The preferred volume of injection is 0.1 ml. Different suspension media can be used to suspend the tumor cells for injection. The commonly used solutions are 10% Fetal Bovine Serum (FBS) [15] and Madrigal [18]. The use of matrigel as a suspension solution has been helpful because it has shown improved tumor implantation. Matrigel is a liquid when kept in low temperature and acquires a gel form when exposed to body temperature. Matrigel contains extracellular matrix components such as laminin and collagen IV, tumor growth factors such as transforming growth factor beta, fibroblast growth factor, and tissue plasminogen activator. These components aid in implantation of the human tumor cells [18].

The resultant tumor can be followed easily and the growth can be monitored accurately as the tumor is on the outer surface of the mouse's body (Figure 1- showing a medium sized tumor on flank of a mouse). Also the tumor can grow to a substantial size without causing much discomfort to the animal.

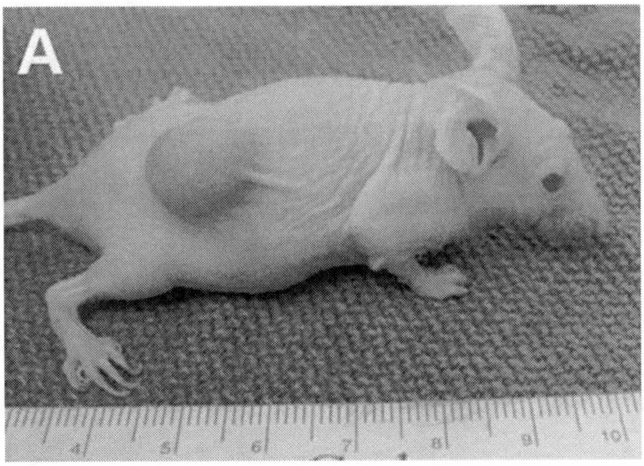

Figure 1. A heterotropic tumor on the flank of a mouse.

Making a heterotopic model may be easy, but it has multiple drawbacks. The use of these models is limited by the fact that it does not mimic the human disease process because of its extra - anatomic site of tumor growth. Also, the absence of metastasis from the subcutaneous site renders the model inappropriate for investigating the spontaneous metastatic process [15].

One of the present uses of the heterotopic model is as a step for making the orthotopic model. The subcutaneously grown tumor is resected after euthanizing the animal and small parts of the tumor are then implanted in the colon to make the orthotopic model [19].

2. Orthotopic Models

Orthotopic tumor models were initially developed utilizing injection of CRC tumor cells or implantation of tumor tissue in the cecum. Such models have been found to be relevant in portraying the human metastatic process [20-23]. Tumors grown orthotopically also have different sensitivities to chemotherapy as compared to heterotopic tumors [24]. Thus the orthotopic techniques provide a complementary tool that enables the study of spontaneous tumor metastasis in a model resembling the human CRC.

While commercially available cell lines can be used for making the orthotopic tumors, implanting or injecting material directly from patient's tumors has also been performed which made it possible to study tumors that have not been altered by years of culture in vitro.

One of the initial orthotopic model creation techniques utilized an open operation. This technique required general anesthesia to the mouse and post operative analgesics. A detailed procedure of the open implantation technique was also described by Pocard and colleagues [19]. Subcutaneous xenografts are made initially by injection of $1X10^6$ tumor cells subcutaneously in the flanks of the mice. When the subcutaneous tumors attain a size of >1 cm^3, the mouse is euthanized and the tumor is cut into pieces measuring 2X2X2 mm. Superficial regions of the tumors are used for implantation and all sampled tumors should be examined histologically to confirm that areas of the tumor correspond to the sampled regions containing viable tumor tissue. Under anesthesia a midline abdominal incision is made and the peritoneal cavity is entered. The cecum is identified and exteriorized through the incision, and a piece of tumor tissue is sutured to the cecal surface with a single Maxon 7/0 stitch, leaving the tumor tissue buried in a 'pouch' consisting of a double cecal wall on each side. After implantation, the abdominal wall is closed in two layers and skin edges are approx.-imated with tissue glue.

A similar model can also be made by injecting the grown tumor cells directly into the submucosal layer of colonic wall from the serosal side at the cecum or the rectum under direct vision [22,25,26]. All other operative steps remain the same as mentioned above except for the tumor cell injection in place of the tumor tissue being implanted.

There are multiple drawbacks of the open orthotopic models as the initial immune response following the surgical model limits the feasibility and reliability of future research goals of monitoring the immune response following open and minimally invasive colorectal resection. Also, the surgical orthotopic implantation model in nude mice does not generate mesenteric and retroperitoneal lymphatic metastases [27]. Moreover these models require the previous expansion of the tumor in subcutaneous xenografts [15,28], which have shown to alter the cell line's growth and dissemination capability [29].

An orthotopic implantation murine model of rectal carcinoma was reported by Takahashi and associates [30]. They reported a technique in which male BALB/c mice were fed a diet containing 3% dextran sulfate sodium (DSS) for seven days to induce colitis and CRC cells were infused intrarectally. They reported a tumor incidence of 94% at 4 weeks of tumor cell instillation. Also the tumor was formed initially at the rectal mucosa at 1 week and then became invasive into the submucosa and muscular tissues at 3 weeks after implantation.

The DSS model of CRC also was evaluated by Clapper and colleagues [31]. They reported that the cyclical administration of DSS in drinking water resulted in the establishment of chronic colitis and the development of colorectal dysplasias and CRC with pathological features resembling human colitis associated neoplasia. The incidence and multiplicity of lesions observed varies depending on the mouse strain used (ie, Swiss Webster, C57BL/6J, CBA, ICR) and the dose (0.7% - 5.0%) and the schedule (1 - 15 cycles with or without a subsequent recovery period) of DSS. Also the incidence of the neoplasia can be increased along with its progression to invasive CRC by administering DSS in combination with a known CRC carcinogen (azoxymethane (AOM), 2- amino-3-methylimidazo{4,5-fl} quinoline (IQ), 2-amino-1-methyl-6-phenylimidazo [4,5-b] pyridine (PhIP)) or iron.

Donigan and colleagues reported a non - operative injection murine model of rectal carcinoma [32] in which the CRC cells were injected into the rectal wall of the mouse under magnification. They reported a tumor 'take' rate of 43% with the use of 10X magnification and an 80% 'take' rate with 100X magnification and an overall 'take' rate of 65%.

Although the model is made with a minimally invasive technique, the essential drawback remains that the injection of the cells into the rectal wall results in tumors not originating from the mucosa.

Using the similar concept of tumor cell injection into the colonic wall, Zigmond and colleagues reported a murine model in which the injection was done through the murine colonoscope (Coloview- Karl Storz) [33].

Overcoming the problems and limitations with the previously described CRC murine models, a true orthotopic murine model using implantation after low-dose colonic mucosal coagulation, followed by transanal instillation of CRC cell lines was reported [18]. Under anesthesia, mice were subjected to low dose electrocoagulation of the colonic mucosa through a transanally inserted small electrode, which was followed by instillation of the CRC tumor cells transanally. As the electrocoagulation was of a low dose, the mucosal injury was limited, and the subsequently instilled tumor cells implanted on the injured mucosa and proliferated in the non-ischemic bed. The resultant tumors grew from the mucosal surface and subsequently involved the deeper colonic layers. Coloview can be used to confirm tumor growth and follow up of these tumors [18,33]. The colonoscopic view of the normal mouse colon shows a smooth circumferential mucosa, so the orthotopically grown tumor from the mucosal surface can be easily detected and followed (Figure 2).

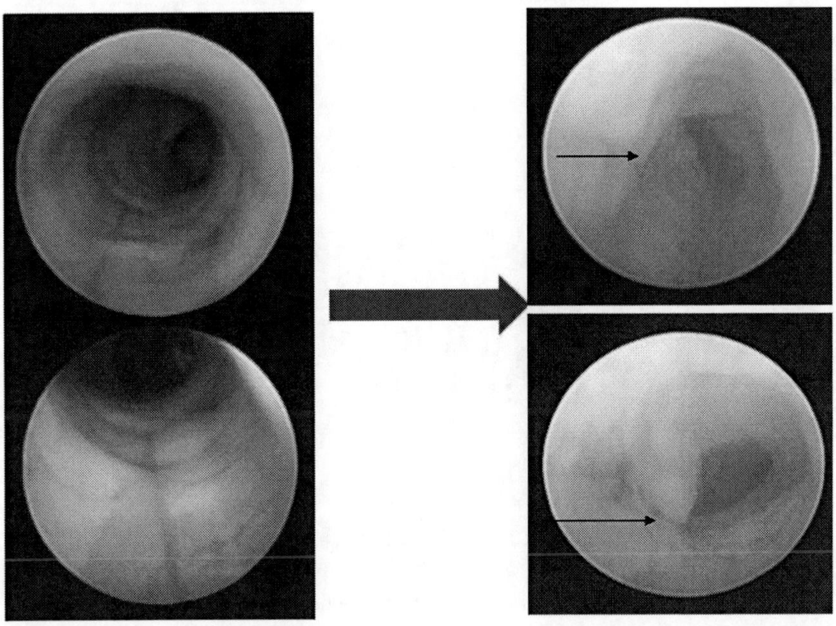

Figure 2. Colonoscopic pictures on the left show a normal murine colon with smooth circumferential mucosa. Colonoscopic pictures on the right shows orthotopic tumor growth in a murine colon (Arrows).

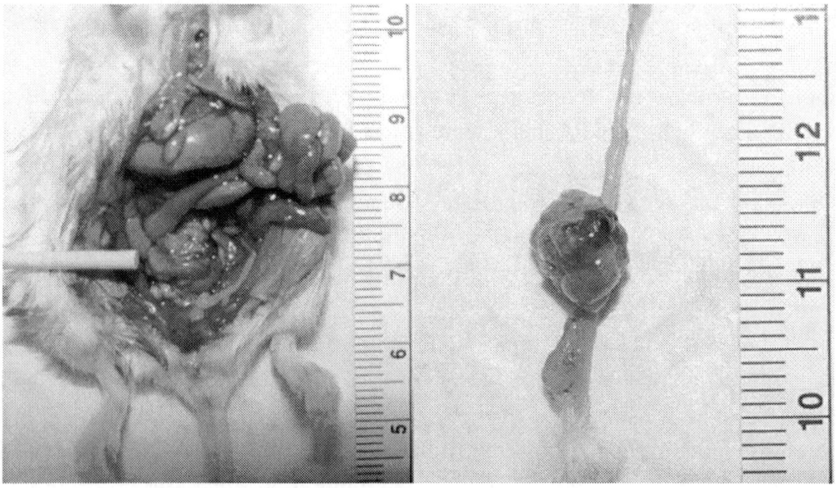

Figure 3. The wood stick points to a colon tumor *in situ* (left) and the dissected colon tumor (right).

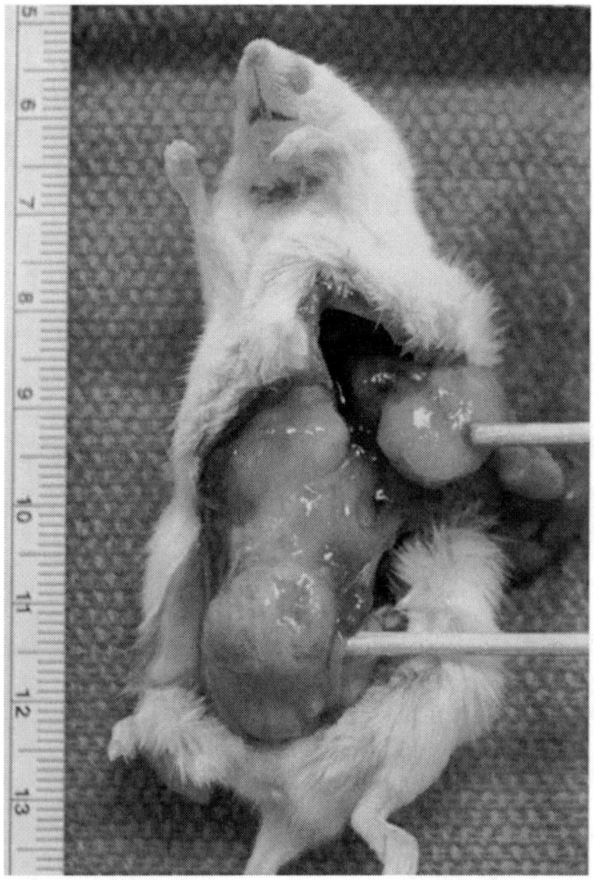

Figure 4. Large orthotopic CRC involving the surrounding structures (Lower wood stick), along with a metastatic matted group of lymph nodes (Upper wood stick).

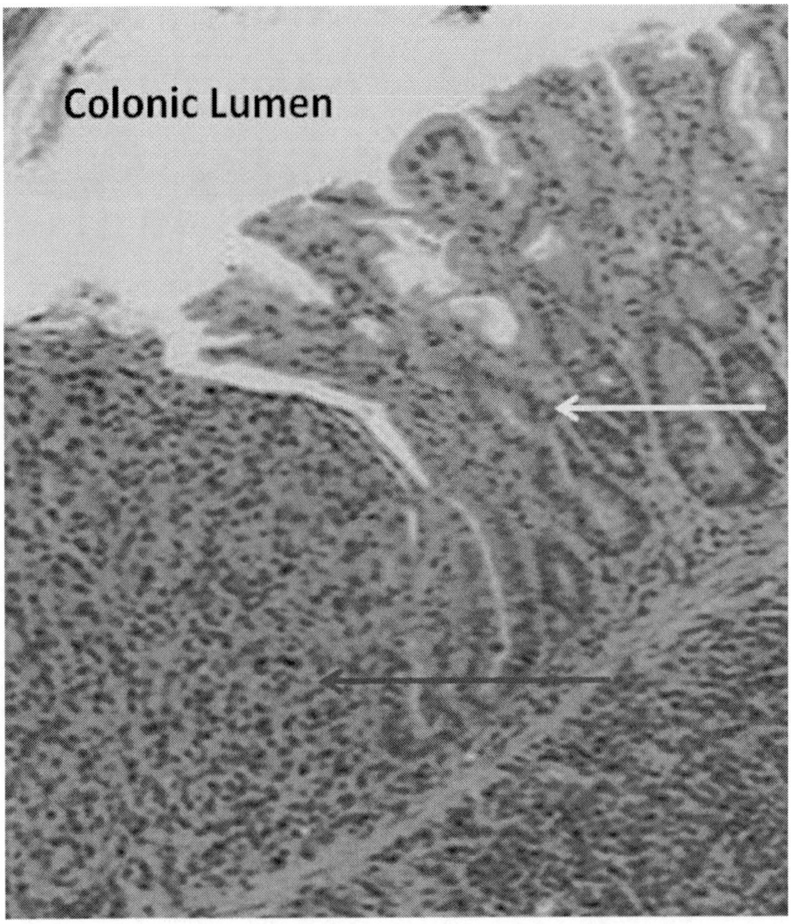

Figure 5. (H &E, 100 X) Orthotopic colon tumor growing on the colon mucosal surface (black arrow), surrounded by normal colon mucosa (white arrow).

Tumors successfully grew in 12 of 12 and 11 of 12 mice with murine tumor lines (CRL-2638 and CRL 2639, respectively) and in 7 of 12 and 12 of 12 mice with human tumor lines (HT-29 and LS 174T, respectively). The tumors were initially smaller (Figure 3), but over time grew larger to invade the surrounding structures such as the bladder, pelvic bones, etc (Figure 4). Histologic evaluation revealed that these tumors grew from the mucosal lining (Figure 5). Metastatic disease was also detected in all of the cell lines (Figure 6). This model overcame the prior limitations such as the variables arising from the need for laparotomy to establish tumor implantation and may allow for better studies in a biologically equivalent animal model of CRC behavior in humans.

Conclusion

As more investigative research continues into the pathology and therapeutic interventions of CRC, the murine model of human CRC will continue to play an essential role. The latest murine models accurately represent and reproduce the human disease process. With better understanding of the disease process combined with the improved technology available to future researchers, we can expect more advancements in the treatment of CRC, directly attributed to the utilization of the murine models of human CRC.

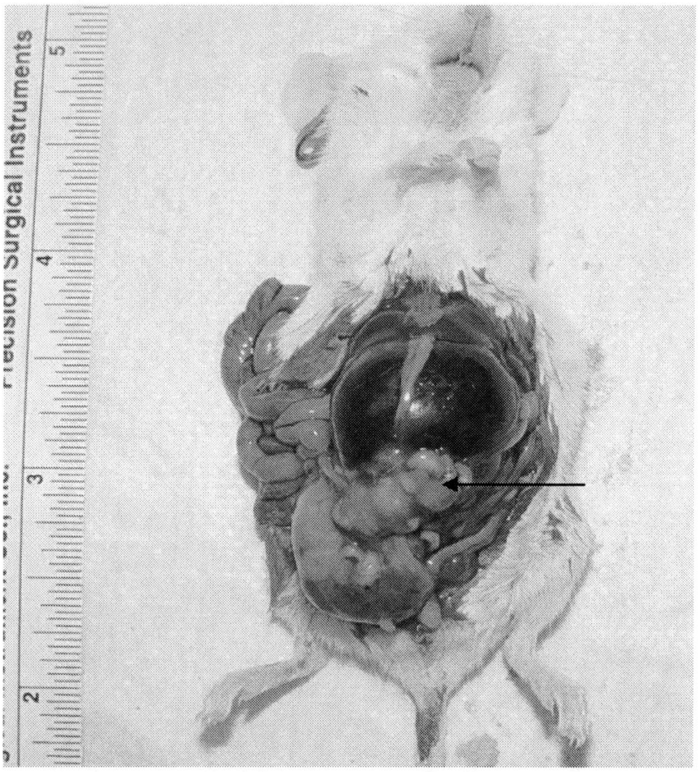

Figure 6. The black arrow points to massive liver metastasis from the orthotopic CRC. The remaining normal liver is displaced upwards. The colon tumor with local invasion into the surrounding tissues is apparent in the right lower quadrant of the abdomen.

References

[1] Taketo MM, Edelmann W. Mouse models of colon cancer. *Gastroenterology* 2009,136: 780–798.

[2] Hawk ET, Levin B. Colorectal cancer prevention. *J Clin Oncol* 2005, 23(2), 378–391.

[3] Theodora Voskoglou-Nomikos, Joseph L. Pater, and Lesley Seymour. Clinical Predictive Value of the *in Vitro* Cell Line, Human Xenograft, and Mouse Allograft Preclinical Cancer Models. *Clinical Cancer Research. Vol. 9*, 4227–4239, September 15, 2003.

[4] Shoemaker R H., Monks., Alley MC, Scudiero D A, Fine D L, McLemore T L, Abbott B J, Paull K D, Mayo JG, and Boyd MR. Development of human tumor cell line panels for use in disease-oriented drug screening. *Prog. Clin. Biol. Res.*, 276: 265–286, 1988.

[5] Skehan P, Storeng R, Scudiero D, Monks A, McMahon J, Vistica D, Warren JT, Bokesch H, Kenney S, and Boyd MR. New colorimetric cytotoxicity assay for anticancer drug screening. *J. Natl. Cancer Inst.* (Bethesda), 82: 1107–1112, 1990.

[6] Rubinstein LV, Shoemaker RH, Paull KD, Simon RM, Tosini S, Skehan P, Scudiero D, Monks A, and Boyd M R. Comparison of *in vitro* anticancer drug screening data generated with a tetrazolium assay *versus* a protein assay against a diverse panel of human tumor cell lines. *J. Natl. Cancer Inst.* (Bethesda), 82*:* 1113–1118, 1990.

[7] Johnson JI, Decker S, Zaharevitz D, Rubinstein LV, Venditti J M., Schepartz S, Kalyandrug S, Christin M, Arbuck S, Hollingshead M, and Sausville EA. Relationships between drug activity in NCI preclinical *in vitro* and *in vivo* models and early clinical trials. *Br. J. Cancer*, 84*:* 1424–1431, 2001.

[8] Venditti J M. The National Cancer Institute antitumor drug discovery program, current and future perspectives: a commentary. *Cancer Treat. Rep.*, 67*:* 767–772, 1983

[9] Zubrod CG. Chemical control of cancer. *Proc. Natl. Acad. Sci. USA*, 69*:* 1042–1047, 1972.

[10] Marsoni S, Hoth D, Simon R, Leyland-Jones B, De Rosa M, and Wittes RE. Clinical drug development: an analysis of Phase II trials, 1970–1985. *Cancer Treat. Rep.*1987, 71*:* 71–80.

[11] Denis E. Corpet, Fabrice Pierre. How good are rodent models of carcinogenesis in predicting efficacy in humans? A systematic review and meta-analysis of colon chemoprevention in rats, mice and men. *European Journal of Cancer* 41 (2005) 1911–1922.

[12] Reichling T, Goss KH, Carson DJ, et al. Transcriptional profiles of intestinal tumors in Apc (Min) mice are unique from those of embryonic intestine and identify novel gene targets dysregulated in human colorectal tumors. *Cancer Res* 2005, 65(1), 166–176.

[13] Edelmann L, Edelmann W. Loss of DNA mismatch repair function and cancer predisposition in the mouse: animal models for human hereditary nonpolyposis colorectal cancer. *American journal of medical genetics Part C, Seminars in medical genetics* 129C: 91–99.

[14] Moser AR, Pitot HC, Dove WF.A dominant mutation that predisposes to multiple intestinal neoplasia in the mouse. *Science* 247: 322–324.

[15] Flatmark K, Maelandsmo GM, Martinsen M, Rasmussen H, Fodstad Ø. Twelvecolorectalcancercelllinesexhibithighlyvariablegrowth and metastatic capacities in an orthotopic model in nude mice. *Eur J Cancer.*2004 Jul;40(10):1593-8.

[16] Kuo TH, Kubota T, Watanabe M, et al. Liver colonization competence governs colon cancer metastasis. *Proc Natl Am Soc USA* 1995, 92, 12085–12089.

[17] Fodstad O. Transplantability of Human Tumors in Nude Mice. *The Nude Mouse in Oncology*. Amsterdam, CRC Press, 1991. 65–88.

[18] Bhullar JS, Subhas G, Silberberg B, Tilak J, Andrus L, Decker M, Mittal VK. A novel nonoperative orthotopic colorectal cancer murine model using electrocoagulation.*J Am Coll Surg*. 2011 Jul;213(1):54-60; discussion 60-1.

[19] Pocard M, Tsukui H, Salmon RJ, et al. Efficiency of orthotopic xenograft models for human colon cancers. *In Vivo* 1996, 10, 463–469.

[20] Fu XY, Besterman JM, Monosov A, et al. Models of human metastatic colon cancer in nude mice orthotopically constructed by using histologically intact patient specimens. *Proc Natl Am Soc USA* 1991, 88, 9345–9349.

[21] Giavazzi R, Campbell DE, Jessup JM, et al. Metastatic behavior of tumor cells isolated from primary and metastatic human colorectal carcinomas implanted into different sites in nude mice. *Cancer Res* 1986, 46, 1928–1933.

[22] Morikawa K, Walker SM, Nakajima M, et al. Influence of organ environment on the growth, selection, and metastasis of human colon carcinoma cells in nude mice. *Cancer Res* 1988, 48, 6863–6871.

[23] Fidler IJ. Critical factors in the biology of human cancer metastasis: twenty-eighth G.H.A. Clowes memorial award lecture. *Cancer Res* 1990, 50, 6130–6138.

[24] Wilmanns C, Fan D, O'Brian CA, et al. Orthotopic and ectopic organ environments differentially influence the sensitivity of murine colon carcinoma cells to doxorubicin and 5-fluorouracil. *Int J Cancer* 1992, 52, 98–104.

[25] Bresalier RS, RAper SE, Hujanen ES, Kim YS. A new animal model for human colon cancer metastasis. *Int J Cancer* 1987;39:625-30.

[26] Tsutsumi S, Kuwano H, Morinaga N, Shimura T, Asao T. Animal model of para-aortic lymph node metastasis. *Cancer Lett* 2001;169:77-85.

[27] Rashidi B, Gamagami R, Sasson A, et al. An orthotopic mouse of remetastasis of human colon cancer liver metastasis. *Clin Cancer Res* 2000;6:2556-2561.

[28] Guibaud N, Kraus-Berthier L, Meyer- Losic F, et al. A marked antitumor activity of a new potent acronycine device in orthotopic models of human solid tumors. *Clin Cancer Res* 2001;7:2573-2580.

[29] Farre L, Casanova I, Guerrero S, et al. Heterotropic implantation alters the regulation of apoptosis and the cell cycle and generates a new metastatic site in human pancreatic tumor xenograft model. *FASEB J* 2001;16:975-982.

[30] Takahashi T, Morotomi M, Nomoto K. A novel mouse model of rectal cancer established by orthotopic implantation of colon cancer cells. *Cancer Sci* 2004;95:514-519.

[31] Margie Lee Clapper, Harry Stanley Cooper and Wen-Chi Lee Chang. Dextran sulfate sodium - induces colitis - associated neoplasia: a promising model for the development of chemopreventive interventions. *Acta Pharmacol Sin* 2007Sep;28(9):1450-1459.

[32] Melissa Donigan, Laurie S Norcross, John Aversa, Jimmie Colon, Joshua Smith, Rafael Madero - Visbal, Shuan LI, Neal McCollum, Andrea Ferrara, Joseph T Gallagher and Cheryl H Baker. Novel murine model for colon cancer: Non - operative trans - anal rectal injection. *Journal of Surgical research* 154 (2009), 299-303.

[33] Ehud Zigmond, Zamir Halpern, Eran Elinav, Eli Brazowski, Steffen Jung and Chen Varol. Utilization of murine colonoscopy for orthotopic implantation of colorectal cancer. *Plos One6*(12): e28858. doi 10.1371/journal.pone.0028858.

Reviewer: The manuscript was reviewed and edited by William C. Cirocco MD, FASCRS, Department of Colorectal Surgery, St. John Van Elslander Cancer Institute, Gross Pointe Woods, MI – 48236, USA.

In: Animal Models in Cancer Research ...
Editor: Sean A. Murray

ISBN: 978-1-62417-587-9

Commentary

Development of Columnar-Lined Esophagus with or without Goblet Cells in Rat Duodenogastroesophageal Reflux Models through Gut Regenerative Cell Lineage (GRCL)

Ken-ichi Mukaisho*[*] *and Takanori Hattori
Depertment of Pathology, Shiga University of Medical Science,
Seta Tukinowa-cho, Otsu, Shiga, Japan

Abstract

Previous studies have focused on goblet cells as the primary marker for Barrett's esophagus (BE), however, recently non-goblet cells, which are columnar-lined esophageal cells resembling gastric cardia-type mucosa, have also been used to define this disease. On the basis of results using rat gastroduodenal contents reflux models, many groups have demonstrated that BE-originating cells are derived from the transcommitment of the esophageal squamous progenitor cells. However, two different lines of evidence have been reported that challenge the transcommitment hypothesis. One is that a discrete population of residual embryonic cells, existing at the gastroesophageal junction in normal individuals, expands and migrates into the esophageal epithelium. The other is that BE originates from gastric cardia progenitors. Recently, we were able to induce cardia-type mucosa without goblet cells in a novel rat reflux model that mimics the human gastroduodenal reflux mechanism. In this the cardia-type mucosa originated not from cells located in the basal layer of the squamous epithelium but from the glandular stomach site. The cardia-type mucosa may progress to specialized intestinal metaplasia (SIM) following continuous bile acids exposure.

[*] Correspondence to: K. Mukaisho, Department of Pathology, Shiga University of Medical Science, Seta-tsukinowa-cho, Otsu, Shiga, 520-2192, Japan, Tel: +81 77 548 2167, Fax: +81 77 543 9880, e-mail: mukaisho @belle.shiga-med.ac.jp.

The concentration and composition of bile acids in the reflux contents may be important factors to decide the pathway and phenotypic switch from gastric to intestinal. We found a peculiar metaplastic change and propose the concept GRCL:Gut regenerative cell lineage (GRCL) develops in response to chronic inflammation. This change is characterized by pyloric–foveolar metaplasia followed by the appearance of goblet cells. SIM also develops through GRCL.

Keywords: Barrett's esophagus, specialized intestinal metaplasia, cardia-type mucosa, GRCL, bile acids

Definition of Barrett's Esophagus

Barrett's esophagus (BE) is defined in the United States (US) by the Practice Parameters Committee of the American College of Gastroenterology as a metaplastic change of the esophageal epithelium of any length that can be recognised at endoscopy and is confirmed by biopsy of the tubular esophagus to have specialised intestinal metaplasia (SIM), excluding intestinal metaplasia of the gastriccardia [1, 2]. Whereas attention in the past has been focused on goblet cells as the primary marker for BE and goblet cells are still generally used to make a formal diagnosis of BE in the US, the recent change in the definition to include non-goblet, columnar lined esophagus resembling cardia-type mucosa was made to acknowledge the more variable histologic presentation of BE in other countries [3-6].

Hypotheses Regarding the Origin of Barrett's Esophagus

A major unanswered question that has been debated for decades is the origin of BE cells. The current hypothesis is that BE originates from the transcommitment of esophageal stem cells to produce an intestine-type epithelium. This hypothesis has been developed from results of animal experiments, but such a transcommitment phenomenon is limited in empirical data from human BE samples. Two recent interesting lines of evidence challenge this prevailing concept of the transcommitment of esophageal stem cells. One is that a discrete population of residual embryonic cells (RECs), existing at the gastroesophageal junction in normal individuals, expands and colonizes regions of the esophagus denuded by chronic reflux [7, 8]. The other is that BE originates from gastric cardia progenitors present in the squamo-columnar junction. The development of these lesions is accelerated by bile acids exposure and nitrosamines [9]. We are planning to check these possibilities in our animal experiments in future.

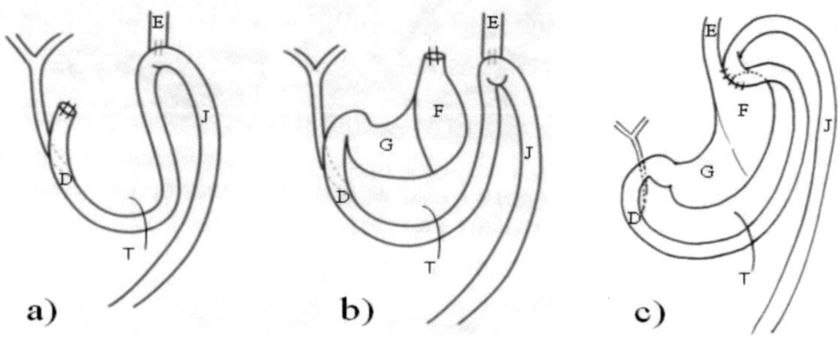

Figure 1. Previous duodenal contents reflux models, E: Esophagus, D: Duodenum; F: Forestomach; G: Glandular stomach; J: Upper jejunum; T: Treitz ligament. a)Esophago-jejunal anastomosis after total gastrectomy [ref. 11]., b) Esophago-jejunal anastomosis without gastrectomy [ref. 10]., c) Esophago-gastro-jejunal anastomosis [ref. 14]. Direct connection between the esophagus and jejunum were made in all animal models.

Rat Gastroduodenal Contents Reflux Models

A Novel Reflux Model

To study the histogenesis of BE and esophageal adenocarcinoma (EAC), several rat gastroduodenal contents reflux models have been developed (Fig. 1) [10-13]. However, gastroduodenal or duodenal contents reflux in these rat models may differ from human acid and duodenal contents reflux because of differences in the esophagogastric junction, except in cases of reconstruction after total gastrectomy. Until recently, many groups, including ours, have used these models to demonstrate that the cell origin in BE originates from progenitor cells in the esophagus. To make clear the differences between rat and human and to clarify the histogenesis of columnar-lined esophagus developing in esophagogastric junction, we recently designed a novel rat gastroduodenal contents reflux model that mimics the human acid and duodenal contents reflux mechanism through a neo-glandular stomach-esophageal stoma (Fig. 2). We studied the histogenesis of columnar metaplasia developed in the anastomosis between the esophagus and glandular stomach after following surgery. We used 8-week-old male Wistar rats weighing approximately 250 g, and a midline laparotomy incision was made under inhalation general anesthesia. The forestomach was removed because human does not have forestomach consisting of squamous epithelium. And the esophagus was cut about 5 mm longitudinally to destroy the lower sphincter of esophagus. The esophagus was connected with the glandular stomach after matching the size of the cut end of the glandular stomach (Figs. 2a–2c). This procedure could induce back flow of all duodenal contents into the glandular stomach was made (Figs. 2d and 2e). As a result, gastric juice, including duodenal contents, flowed to the esophagus through the neo-glandular stomach-esophageal stoma (Figs. 2e) [14]. The procedure of operation is very complicated and it takes about 1.5h. And survival rate was about 60%. However, if the operation is succeeded, the animal can survive for long duration. At 50 weeks after reflux surgery, cardia-type mucosa without goblet cells was observed at the neo-esophago-glandular stomach junction (Fig. 3a). The cardia-type mucosa occurred from the glandular stomach site and was composed of cells positively for MUC5AC (gastric foveolar-type mucin, 45M1, Thermo) in the surface mucosa and for HIK1083 (gastric pyloric gland-type mucin, HIK1083, Kanto Chem) at the base (Figs. 3b and 3c). The developing process of these cardia-type mucosa in the recent model seems to be "regeneration" to repair ulcer lesion arising in the neo-esophago-glandular stomach junction. Neither dysplasia nor adenocarcinoma was detected for up to 50 weeks after surgery. However, a few cells positive for a caudal-related homeobox intestinal transcription factor CDX2 (CDX2-88, BioGenex) were occasionally detected in the cardia-type mucosa (Figs. 3d) [14].

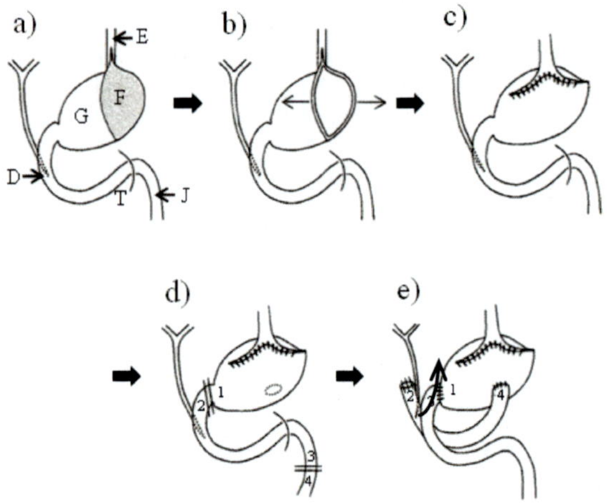

Figure 2. Surgical procedure. E: Esophagus, D: Duodenum; F: Forestomach; G: Glandular stomach; J: Upper jejunum; T: Treitz ligament. All duodenal contents flow back into the glandular stomach through the gastrojejunal stoma. As a result, gastric juice, including duodenal contents, flow to the esophagus through the gastroesophageal stoma (arrow in Figure 2e).

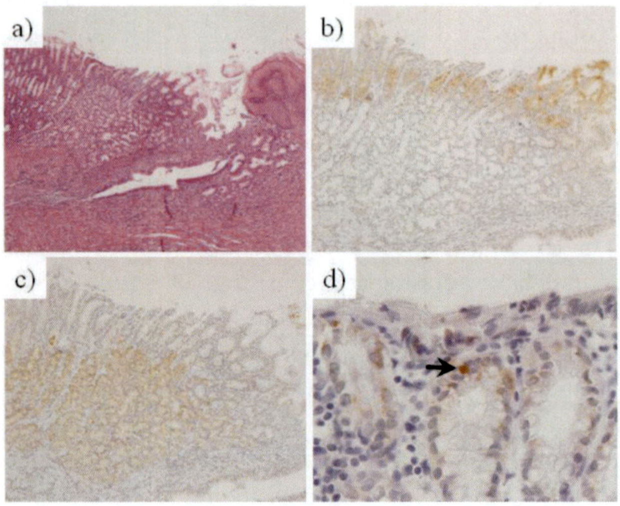

Figure 3. Cardiac-type mucosa developed in the novel animal model. a) Hematoxylin and eosin staining, b)MUC5AC, c)HIK1083, d) CDX2. a)Proliferation of cardia-type glands occurs from the normally present gastriccardia-type mucosa in the regeneration process. b) and c) The metaplastic glands were stained positively for MUC5AC in the surface mucosa and for HIK1083 at the base, respectively. d) A few CDX2-positive cells are occasionally detected in the cardia-type mucosa (arrow).

Previous Reflux Models

In previous studies of the animal models, the columnar-lined esophagus developed in the form of SIM with well-developed goblet cells. SIM developed at about 20 weeks after reflux surgery, and EAC was noted at 30–40 weeks after reflux surgery [10-13]. SIM mainly originated from cells located in the basal layer of the esophageal squamous epithelium (Fig. 4a). One of the important points is that buds of this SIM had cells positive for gastric type mucins [13, 14]. And the full-brown SIM with goblet cells positive for MUC2 (H-300, Santa Cruz) (Fig. 4b) often had partly the cells with gastric type mucins [14]. Moreover the pyloric-type glands positive for HIK1083 were found to be located at the bottom of SIM (Fig. 4c). These glands were different from the proper pyloric glands, because these glands had cells positive for CDX2 (Fig. 4d) [14, 15]. Proliferation of pyloric-type glands was also occasionally seen in parts of esophagojejunal anastomosis in previous models (Fig. 5). This finding suggests that BE progenitor cells may also develop from jejunnal crypt, because there was no connection between glandular stomach and esophagus. This phenomenon may be explained by a hypothesis, which Xian et al. proposed, that RECs are distributed throughout the upper gastrointestinal tract [8].

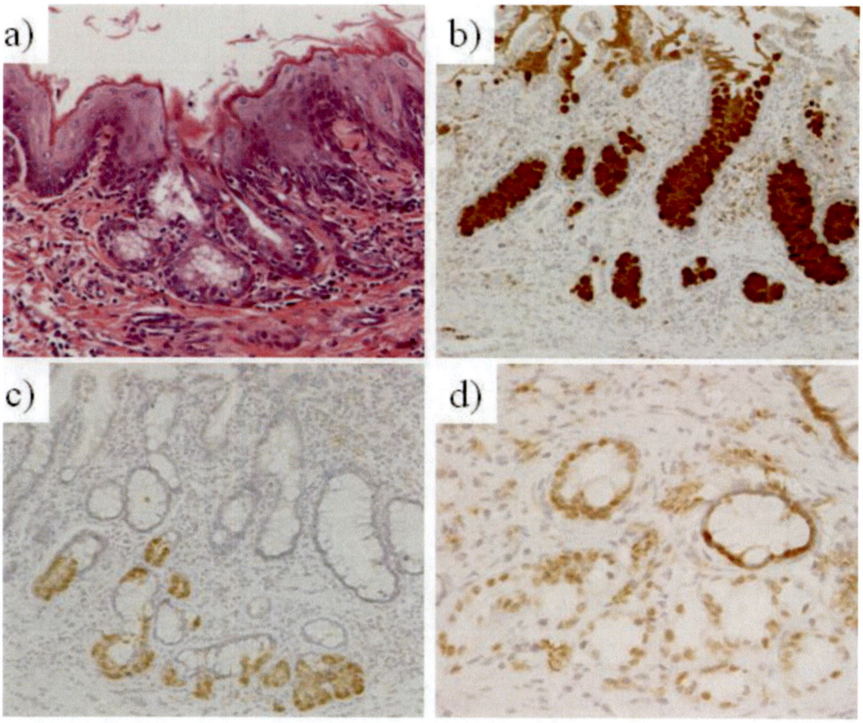

Figure 4. Histological findings of specialized intestinal metaplasia (SIM) a) Hematoxylin and eosin staining, b)MUC2, c)HIK1083, d)CDX2. SIM with goblet cells was detected in previous animal models of esophagojejunostomy. SIM was derived from transdifferentiation of probable stem cells located in the basal layer of the esophageal squamous cell epithelium. b)SIM was positive for MUC2. C) SIM has partly gastric type glands positive for HIK1083 at the bottom of glands. d) The pyloric-type glands are positive for CDX2.

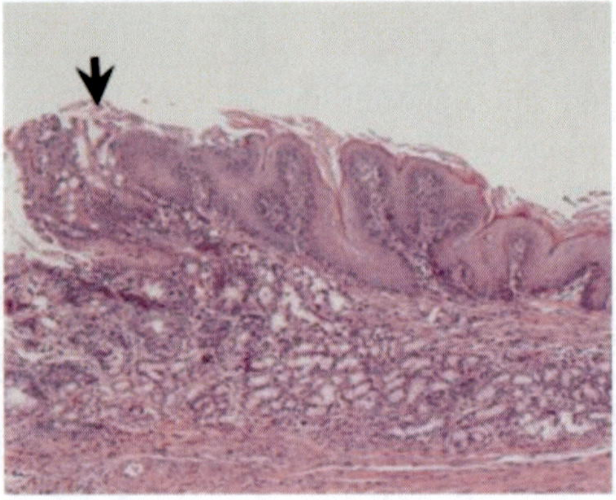

Figure 5 Proliferation of pyloric-type glands at the neo-esophago-jejunal junction in previous models. (Right is oral side and left is anal side. An arrow stands for anastomosis.) Pyloric-type glands are developed from the jejunal site.

Dissimilarities between in the Recent Study and in the Previous Study

There seem to be big differences between in the recent model and in the previous models. The former reported that cardiac-type mucosa originated from the normally-present gastric cardia mucosa, and the latter reported that SIM mainly originated from cells located in the basal layer of the esophageal squamous epithelium. This difference may be caused by the differences in concentration of bile acids in the reflux contents. The esophagus in the previous models was exposed to a much higher concentration of duodenal contents, including bile juice, compared with the esophagus in the recent model. This was because the esophagus was directly connected to the intestine in the previous models. Bile acids have been reported to induce overexpression of CDX1 and CDX2 in esophageal epithelium [16, 17]. CDX1 and CDX2 play important roles in the induction and maintenance of SIM [15-17]. On the other hand, there is a report that *Cdx2*-transgenic mice have been reported to develop intestinal-type adenocarcinoma at an age >80 weeks [18]. Intestinal metaplasia itself is now believed to be related to the genesis and progression of gastric carcinoma [18]. Therefore, bile acids that cause overexpression of CDX2, play a role in goblet cell development and EAC carcino-genesis. The other important thing to decide the phenotype of BE may be the bile-acid composition of bile juice in reflux contents. We reported that administration of high animal fat diet caused a change of the bile acid composition as revealed as the increase of taurine conjugates, and it appeared that these changes promoted the development of BE and Barrett's dysplasia leading to EAC [19].

There are also similarities between in the recent model and in the previous models. The cardia-type mucosa seen in the former model had cells positive for pyloric gland-type mucin. And either BE progenitor cells which occasionally developed in the esophagojejunal stoma in the former model orbuds of SIMseen in the latter models, which appeared to originate from esophageal squamous epithelium had also pyloric gland-type mucin. These pyloric gland-type glands seem to have developed in early phase of regeneration against chronic reflux damage.

A Novel Gut Regenerative Cell Lineage (GRCL) Theory

By previous experiments using rat gastroduodenal contents reflux models, we found a peculiar metaplastic change leading to development of SIM and we proposed the concept of gut regenerative cell lineage (GRCL) theory. GRCL occurs during the regenerative process in response to chronic inflammation (Fig. 6) [12-15, 20]. This change is characterized by pyloric–foveolar metaplasia followed by the appearance of goblet cells [12-15, 20]. In addition, the expression of both CDX1 and CDX2 was found to play a crucial role in directing intestinal-type differentiation of GRCL [12, 14, 15]. The occurrence of such pyloric–foveolar metaplasia has been reported frequently in the entire gut, and this phenol-menon is described as aberrant pyloric glands or pseudopyloric metaplasia in cases of Crohn's disease [21], pseudopyloric gland metaplasia of the fundic stomach with chronic gastritis [22], gastrointestinal metaplasia of gallbladder with chronic cholecystitis [23], gastric metaplasia in duodenal ulcers [24], and colonic dysplasia following ulcerative colitis [25]. We also suggested that GRCL is related to intestinal-type carcinogenesis (Fig. 6) [12-15, 20]. In the course of the animal experiments using the recent model, we detected a few CDX2-positive cells in cardia-type mucosa prior to the development of BE or EAC. The columnar-lined metaplasia without goblet cells developed in the recent models may also be included in the development of SIM through GRCL. However, the time required to transform from cardia-type mucosa to SIM may be prolonged in this model.

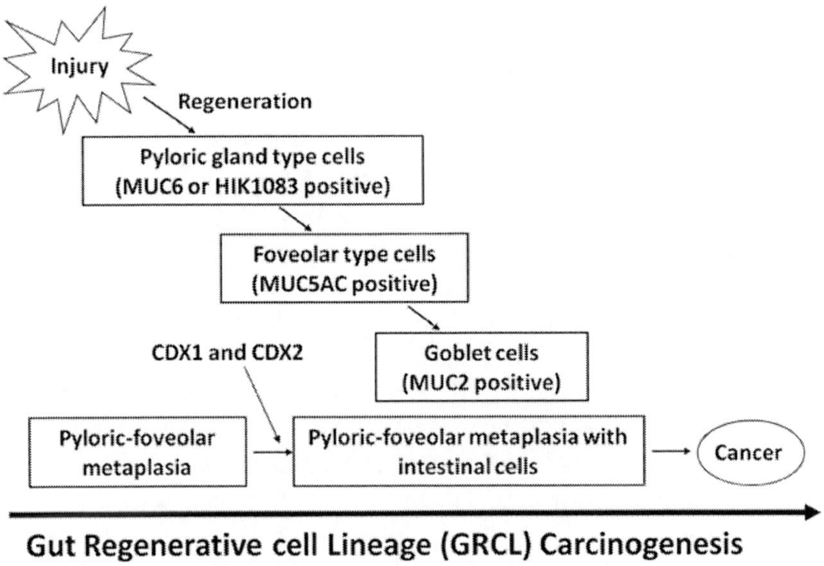

Figure 6. Gut regenerative cell lineage (GRCL) carcinogenesis. The GRCL is characterized by pyloric-foveolar metaplasia with appearance of goblet cells, which occurs in the regenerative process in response to chronic inflammation. A situation is analogous to the incomplete intestinal metaplasia of gastric-intestinal mixed type in the stomach. BE very likely develops through the GRCL, and CDX1 and CDX2 play a crucial role in directing intestinal-type differentiation of the GRCL. GRCL is also related to intestinal-type carcinogenesis.

Taken together, we were able to induce two types of BE. One is cardia-type mucosa in the recent model, which mimics the human gastroduodenal reflux mechanism through a stoma at the neo-esophago-glandular stomach junction. The mucosa originated not from cells located in the basal layer of the squamous epithelium but from the glandular stomach site following regeneration. The cardia-type mucosa may progress to SIM following continuous bile acids exposure. The other is metaplastic development of SIM. The columnar conversion first occurs from probable stem cells located in the basal layer of squamous epithelium. The concentration and composition of bile acids in reflux contents may be a key factor to determine the pathway and phenotypic switch.

References

[1] Spechler SJ. Barrett's esophagus: Clinical issues. *Gastrointest Endosc Clin N Am.* 2011;21:1-7.

[2] Wakelin DE, Al-Mutawa T, Wendel C, Green C, Garewal HS, Fass R.A predictive model for length of Barrett's esophagus with hiatal hernia length and duration of esophageal acid exposure. *Gastrointest Endosc* 2003; 58: 350–5.

[3] Badreddine RJ, Wang KK. Barrett esophagus: an update. *Nat Rev Gastroenterol Hepatol.* 2010;7:369-78.

[4] Playford RJ. New British Society of Gastroenterology (BSG) guidelines for the diagnosis and management of Barrett's oesophagus. *Gut* 2006 ; 55 :442.

[5] Takubo K, Aida J, Naomoto Y, Sawabe M, Arai T, Shiraishi H, Matsuura M, Ell C, May A, Pech O, Stolte M, Vieth M. Cardiac rather than intestinal-type background in endoscopic resection specimens of minute Barrett adenocarcinoma. *Hum Pathol.* 2009;40:65-74.

[6] Riddell RH, Odze RD. Definition of Barrett's esophagus: time for a rethink--is intestinal metaplasia dead? *Am J Gastroenterol.* 2009;104:2588-94.

[7] Wang X, Ouyang H, Yamamoto Y, Kumar PA, Wei TS, Dagher R, Vincent M, Lu X, Bellizzi AM, Ho KY, Crum CP, Xian W, McKeon F. Residualembryoniccells as precursors of a Barrett's-like metaplasia. *Cell.* 2011;145:1023-35.

[8] Xian W, Ho KY, Crum CP, McKeon F. Cellularorigin of Barrett's esophagus: controversy and therapeutic implications. *Gastroenterology.* 2012;142:1424-30.

[9] Quante M, Bhagat G, Abrams JA, Marache F, Good P, Lee MD, Lee Y, Friedman R, Asfaha S, Dubeykovskaya Z, Mahmood U, Figueiredo JL, Kitajewski J, Shawber C, Lightdale CJ, Rustgi AK, Wang TC. Bileacid and inflammationactivate-gastriccardiastemcells in a mousemodel of Barrett-likemetaplasia. *Cancer Cell.* 2012 ;21:36-51.

[10] Fein M, Peters JH, Chandrasoma P, Ireland AP, Oberg S, Ritter MP, Bremner CG, Hagen JA, DeMeester TR. Duodenoesophageal reflux induces esophageal adenocarcinoma without exogenous carcinogen.*J Gastrointest Surg*. 1998;2:260-8.

[11] Miwa K, Sahara H, Segawa M, Kinami S, Sato T, Miyazaki I, Hattori T. Reflux of duodenal or gastro-duodenal contents induces esophageal carcinoma in rats. *Int J Cancer*. 1996;67:269-74.

[12] Macke RA, Nason KS, Mukaisho K, Hattori T, Fujimura T, Sasaki S, Oyama K, Miyashita T, Ohta T, Miwa K, Gibson MK, Zaidi A, Malhotra U, Atasoy A, Foxwell T, Jobe B. Barrett's esophagus and animal models. *Ann N Y Acad Sci.* 2011;1232:392-400.

[13] Kumagai H, Mukaisho K, Sugihara H, Bamba M, Miyashita T, Miwa K, Hattori T. Cell kinetic study on histogenesis of Barrett's esophagus using rat reflux model. *Scand J Gastroenterol.* 2003;38:687-92.

[14] Mukaisho K, Kushima R, Takemura S, Araki Y, Vieth M, Sugihara H, Hattori T. Histogenesis of Barrett's adenocarcinoma: analyses of human samples and results of experimental animal studies. *Stomach and Intestine,* 2011;46: 1861-74, (in Japanese)

[15] Tatsuta T, Mukaisho K, Sugihara H, Miwa K, Tani T, Hattori T. Expression of Cdx2 in early GRCL of Barrett's esophagus induced in rats by duodenal reflux. *Dig Dis Sci.* 2005 50:425-31.

[16] Kazumori H, Ishihara S, Kinoshita Y. Roles of caudal-related homeobox gene Cdx1 in oesophageal epithelial cells in Barrett's epithelium development. *Gut.* 2009;58:620-8.

[17] Burnat G, Rau T, Elshimi E, Hahn EG, Konturek PC. Bile acids induce overexpression of homeobox gene CDX-2 and vascular endothelial growth factor (VEGF) in human Barrett's esophageal mucosa and adenocarcinoma cell line. *Scand J Gastroenterol.* 2007;42:1460-5.

[18] Mutoh H, Sakurai S, Satoh K, Tamada K, Kita H, Osawa H, Tomiyama T, Sato Y, Yamamoto H, Isoda N, Yoshida T, Ido K, Sugano K. Development of gastric carcinoma from intestinal metaplasia in Cdx2-transgenic mice. *Cancer Res.* 2004 ;64:7740-7.

[19] Chen KH, Mukaisho K, Sugihara H, Araki Y, Yamamoto G, Hattori T. High animal-fat intake changes the bile-acid composition of bile juice and enhances the development of Barrett's esophagus and esophageal adenocarcinoma in a rat duodenal-contents reflux model. *Cancer Sci.* 2007;98:1683-8.

[20] Mukaisho K, Miwa K, Kumagai H, Bamba M, Sugihara H, Hattori T. Gastric carcinogenesis by duodenal reflux through gut regenerative cell lineage. *Dig Dis Sci.* 2003;48:2153-8.

[21] Kushima R, Borchard F, Hattori T. A new aspect of gastric metaplasia in Crohn's disease: bidirectional (foveolar and pyloric) differentiation in so-called 'pyloric metaplasia' in the ileum. *Pathol Int.* 1997;47:416-9.

[22] Hattori T, Helpap B, Gedigk P. The morphology and cell kinetics of pseudopyloric glands. *Virchows Arch B Cell Pathol Incl Mol Pathol.* 1982;39:31-40.

[23] Shimizu M, Kitoh K, Fujimitsu Y, Inada K, Ichinose M, Miki K, Yamao K, Nakazawa S, Shamoto M, Tatematsu M. Cellular differentiation and development of pyloric mucosal metaplasia in the human gall-bladder. *Pathol Int.* 1996;46:261-6.

[24] Kushima R, Manabe R, Hattori T, Borchard F. Histogenesis of gastric foveolar metaplasia following duodenal ulcer: a definite reparative lineage of Brunner's gland. *Histopathology.* 1999;35:38-43.

[25] Tatsumi N, Kushima R, Vieth M, Mukaisho K, Kakinoki R, Okabe H, Borchard F, Stolte M, Okanoue T, Hattori T. Cytokeratin 7/20 and mucin core protein expression in ulcerative colitis-associated colorectal neoplasms. *Virchows Arch.* 2006;448:756-62.

Index

D

E

F

G

H

N

O

P

Q

R

S

T

U

V

W

X

Y

Z